Acclaim for Pedro Lemebel and
A Last Supper of Queer Apostles

"[Lemebel] speaks brilliantly for a difference that refuses to disappear."
—Garth Greenwell, *The New Yorker*

"Lemebel doesn't have to write poetry to be the best poet of my generation. . . . When everyone who has treated him like dirt is lost in the cesspit or in nothingness, Pedro Lemebel will still be a star."
—Roberto Bolaño, author of *2666* and *The Savage Detectives*

"If the world were just, Pedro Lemebel would take his rightful place on the throne of literary royalty; although I'm certain he'd reject something as anti-democratic as monarchy. *A Last Supper of Queer Apostles* cements his place in the canon—the literary one, the queer one, the Chilean one, the Latin American one, the human one. This collection of devastatingly gay and unabashedly political essays is, in fact, a quiver of exquisite arrows, each dipped in the blood and bile of love and hate, the only tincture with the viscosity of truth. On every one of these electrifying and gorgeously written pages—brilliantly translated by Gwendolyn Harper—Lemebel spills anti-fascist tea in dizzying prose that spins us ever closer to the collective liberation he was seeking. All hail this queen."
—Alejandro Varela, National Book Award finalist for *The Town of Babylon*

"[Lemebel's writing is] provocative, strange, very Chilean, cantankerous, bitter, funny, sentimental, sharp, elegant, entirely legible and at the same time complex. . . . His work was forged in the night, in the barrio, in life and not in literature. . . . His books changed lives."
—Alejandro Zambra, author of *Multiple Choice* and *Chilean Poet*

"The summary effect of reading Pedro Lemebel's shattering indictment of the American-backed Pinochet regime, of being faced with the caustic rage embedded in it, corresponds to standing transfixed in front of Picasso's *Guernica*, the light bulb eyeball

glaring down at the carnage below, the ocular shriek a fitting match for the illuminating text of *A Last Supper of Queer Apostles*, with its story of death and resurrection."

—James McCourt, author of *Time Remaining* and *Queer Street*

"Lemebel said he writes from difference, and my god, what a difference. His writing is everything except boring—courageous, beautiful, vile, glorious, provocative, comforting, angry, loving, exquisite, and full of delicious venom. Reading a great writer makes life better. Reading Lemebel makes me want to live better."

—Rabih Alameddine, author of *An Unnecessary Woman*

"Reading these powerfully intimate essays makes me feel like I know Pedro Lemebel. His friends are now my friends. The clothes they wore, the way they danced, the way they died—all this will live on in my memory as if I'd always had them in my life."

—Joe Westmoreland, author of *Tramps Like Us*

"A truly astonishing body of work . . . Images so alarming and original leap from every page, you come to believe that if you were to tear a page it would bleed scarlet. . . . The writings of a curbside saint laboring serene under a weight of genius."

—Lauren John Joseph, author of *At Certain Points We Touch*

"A remarkable and radically uncompromising chronicle of queer life in anti-queer times . . . Gwendolyn Harper's translation is astoundingly good. It allowed me to feel that I was being spoken to directly. And to know that Lemebel's personality, his poetry, his love, his grief, his anger, his generosity, his voice, are all still with us, and still true. Pedro Lemebel is alive! And I am in love."

—Keith Ridgway, author of *Hawthorn & Child* and *A Shock*

A LAST SUPPER OF QUEER APOSTLES

PEDRO LEMEBEL (1952–2015) is considered one of the most important queer writers of twentieth-century Latin America and was also an activist and a performance artist. Born in Santiago, Chile, he became a renowned voice of Latin American counterculture during the Pinochet dictatorship and its aftermath. He received Chile's José Donoso Prize and a Guggenheim Fellowship. He is best known for his crónicas and one novel, *My Tender Matador*, which has been translated into more than a dozen languages and was adapted in 2020 into a critically acclaimed film by Chilean director Rodrigo Sepúlveda.

GWENDOLYN HARPER is a writer and a translator of Latin American literature. She won a National Endowment for the Arts fellowship and a Work in Progress grant from the Robert B. Silvers Foundation for *A Last Supper of Queer Apostles*. She holds an MFA from Brown University.

IDRA NOVEY is the award-winning author of the novels *Ways to Disappear*, *Those Who Knew*, and *Take What You Need*. She lived in Chile for several years, returns often, and has translated work by various Chilean writers, including Nona Fernández and Marco Antonio de la Parra. Her own work has been translated into a dozen languages, and she's written for *The Atlantic*, *The New York Times*, and *The Guardian*. She teaches fiction writing at Princeton University.

PEDRO LEMEBEL

A LAST SUPPER OF QUEER APOSTLES

SELECTED ESSAYS

Edited, Translated, and with an Introduction and Notes by
GWENDOLYN HARPER

Foreword by
IDRA NOVEY

PENGUIN BOOKS

PENGUIN BOOKS

An imprint of Penguin Random House LLC
penguinrandomhouse.com

These essays were originally published in Spanish and appeared in *La esquina es mi corazón* (Santiago, Chile: Editoiral Planeta Chilena S.A., 1995), *Loco afán: Crónicas de sidario, 2nd Edition* (Barcelona: Editorial Anagrama, 2000), and *Poco hombre* (Santiago, Chile: Ediciones Universidad Diego Portales, 2013).

LIBRARY OF CONGRESS CATALOGING-IN-PUBLICATION DATA
Names: Lemebel, Pedro, author. | Harper, Gwendolyn, editor, translator, writer of introduction. | Novey, Idra, writer of foreword. | Lemebel, Pedro. Poco hombre. Selections. English. | Lemebel, Pedro. Loco afán. Selections. English. | Lemebel, Pedro. Esquina es mi corazón. Selections. English.
Title: A last supper of queer apostles : selected essays / Pedro Lemebel ; edited, translated, and with an introduction and notes by Gwendolyn Harper ; foreword by Idra Novey.
Description: New York : Penguin Books, 2024. | Includes bibliographical references. |
Identifiers: LCCN 2023053796 (print) | LCCN 2023053797 (ebook) | ISBN 9780143137085 (trade paperback) | ISBN 9780525508588 (ebook)
Subjects: LCSH: Lemebel, Pedro—Translations into English. | LCGFT: Essays.
Classification: LCC PQ8098.22.E57 L37 2024 (print) | LCC PQ8098.22.E57 (ebook) | DDC 864/.64—dc23/eng/20240214
LC record available at https://lccn.loc.gov/2023053796
LC ebook record available at https://lccn.loc.gov/2023053797

Printed in the United States of America
1st Printing

Set in Sabon LT Pro

Contents

COUP

AIDS

POST-90

FINALE

Foreword

Decades ago, I heard an apocryphal story about Pedro Lemebel arriving in a pink miniskirt to receive his first literary prize. I've heard iterations of this story since then from various relatives and friends. It always ends with what he wore, the pink miniskirt serving as cultural shorthand for the far more nuanced insurgency that Lemebel and his writing ignited. It is a liberator tale, marking the arrival of an unforeseen leader, the artist capable of showing all of Chile that performing sameness wasn't as necessary to their survival as they assumed it to be—that they didn't, in fact, need to resign themselves to social and cultural suffocation for the rest of their lives.

The story always takes place in an upper-crust Santiago neighborhood in the early eighties, ten years or so into the Pinochet dictatorship. A well-funded municipality decides to hold a writing contest, with the assumption that only people from nearby households will have the skill and confidence to take their writing seriously enough to submit it. Lemebel grew up not nearby but in one of Santiago's poorest neighborhoods. He submits a poem about the precarity of gay life on the margins of Santiago. Allegedly, several of the judges recoil when they read it, but the images in it are so striking, the language so vivid and exceptional, that they can't deny the truth: the poem merits the prize more than any of the other submissions.

When I researched the veracity of this tale, however, I discovered another story entirely, even more subversive and nuanced. In this version, Lemebel submitted not a poem but a short story about a father who hides his homosexuality from his family.

At that point, Lemebel still used the same first and last name as his father, Pedro Mardones. When someone from the municipal committee arrived with the prize news, Lemebel wasn't home. His father was the one to receive the news at the door, to say yes, he was Pedro Mardones.

A few weeks after reading this version of events on Wikipedia and several other sites, I couldn't find it anywhere, a disappearance that was fitting, as potent with layers of meaning as the extraordinary chronicles of overlooked lives contained in this volume. Lemebel wrote about people who were either caricatured or erased entirely from the public record, people like Silicone María and Our Lady of the Empanada, queens like Coupon, No Guarantees, Seven Asses, and Stick It Up Yours. These crónicas are a testament to the far more varied and beautiful truths about who lives and falls in love in Chile, beyond the fathers that have dominated its literature, with their names that automatically go first on the birth certificates of their children, names that those offspring are expected to keep, which Lemebel did not.

I suspect the story of Lemebel's now legendary entry into Chilean literature will continue to change as the country changes. Óscar Contardo, in his recent biography of Lemebel, *Loca fuerte*, says that Lemebel came to find amusement in the conflicting versions of his life, how they've become a mirror for the country of itself.

What remains an established fact is Lemebel's decision to change, in 1993, his surname to his mother's—a gesture he defined as "an alliance with all that is feminine." I first encountered Lemebel's work around the time I had also dropped my father's last name, upon publication of my first poem, opting instead for a verbal alliance with the Noveys on my mother's side. I was ravenous for writerly gestures of audacity when I arrived in Chile in 2000 for a teaching job at the state-run Catholic University of Valparaíso. A decade had already passed since the 1988 plebiscite ending the dictatorship, but military leaders still oversaw the state university system. The theater productions I went to see in Valparaíso were often inhibited, lacking any genuine daring, or so they seemed until a writer friend invited me to see a series of dramatic monologues based on Lemebel's crónicas. The theater was packed and people were unusually animated, laughing with a contagious sense of excitement.

Once the lone actor stepped onto the stage and began to speak, I lost all interest in the audience. I was stunned. That performance was my first experience of Lemebel's writing, of the verve and endearing idiosyncrasies he grants to each character, of how artfully he juxtaposes the lightness of his sly humor with frank descriptions of the fear, hunger, and efforts at survival that shape the lives of the gender-nonconforming locas in his crónicas. Yet the cruel circumstances in which they live, how many of them die of AIDS with no medical support whatsoever, are never the sum of who they are.

I've now been returning to Lemebel's work for twenty-five years, and each time I learn something new from it about how to write prose with the mindset of a poet, how to subvert conventional ways of describing a character, the subtle gestures that speak to a person's sensuality, the small impulses that reveal their particular way of coping with fear and longing.

Lemebel had a tremendous gift for unexpected metaphors, for how to conjure the singularity of a person through one striking sensual detail. As he writes in one of the indelible crónicas in this volume, "there's always a metaphor that, in ridiculing, beautifies the flaw, making it unique, one's own."

In a now legendary conversation from 2000, TV interviewer Tati Penna describes Lemebel's work as "an acidic vision of our society." With transfixing composure, Lemebel smiles at this description of his work and explains to Penna that when gay people seek a public act, some will inevitably see it as violent, the way, he tells her, "any minority that announces their needs is called violent and disruptive." Lemebel's works are no more acidic than the brutal and often deadly reality in which he wrote them. Throughout the interview, Lemebel insists on the alliance in his work between "homosexuals and other minorities . . . with everyone that Chilean society has denied."

During that TV interview, and for years after and before it, Lemebel described his work with the same four words: "Hablo por mi diferencia." For a writer to speak from, and through, what makes them different may not seem radical now. To speak out of difference has become a more accepted source of artistic vitality in the twenty-first century, or at least in more countries than it used to be, than when Lemebel first entered Chilean literature and was often the only writer determined to make that intention manifest in everything he wrote.

Gwendolyn Harper's lively translations in this volume contain all sorts of inventive re-creations of Lemebel's exacting slices into the intestines of Chilean speech. Lemebel's artful wielding of Chilean slang doesn't lend itself easily to translation. He splits open Chilean Spanish like the underside of a fish, exposing all the slimy cultural guts. Harper's translation attends to all those tacit social connotations in subtle ways. In "Night of Furs," she re-creates the charged humor of Lemebel's cast of locas as they gossip about mainstream TV culture—a culture that has denied their existence. The painful fact of their exclusion flows unspoken beneath their discussion of "handsome Mauricio and his olive-pit pucker" as they egg each other on, exchanging stories about "the kept prince of television." After the joyful banter in the opening pages, "Night of Furs" moves toward the dire torment of "seropositive winters," endured within the ongoing terrors of the dictatorship.

In her deeply considered translations, Harper honors the jarring contrasts "of cadavers and dreams" that Lemebel experienced and transformed into a body of work that deserves a far more prominent place in the international canon of writing that has expanded humanity's understanding of itself. If you have yet to read the work of Pedro Lemebel, prepare to be wrecked and resurrected, to be pulled into the world of characters who come immediately to life and who will not leave you.

My first rapturous encounter with Lemebel's crónicas converged with an early fixation on another South American writer, Clarice Lispector, whose sentences and startling emotional honesty are similarly unmistakable for anyone else's. As with Lispector, whose books have only posthumously been widely recognized as the canonical body of writing that they are, I hope this volume will begin a long overdue international conversation about, and celebration of, Lemebel's exhilarating work.

IDRA NOVEY

Introduction

> I could write almost telegraphically for the whole world and for the symmetrical ratification of all languages kowtowed to English. I'll never write in English; with any luck I say, *Go home.*
>
> —Pedro Lemebel, "In Lieu of a Synopsis"

It's hard to know whether Pedro Lemebel, one of the most important queer writers of twentieth-century Latin America, wants to be translated into English at all after a couple of sentences like that. A protean figure, he was a performance artist, radio host, and newspaper columnist, a tireless activist whose life spanned some of Chile's most dramatic decades. But above all he was known for his furious, dazzling crónicas—short prose pieces that blend loose reportage with fictional and essayistic modes. Many of them depict Chile's AIDS crisis, which in 1984 began to spread through Santiago's sexual underground, overlapping with the final years of the Pinochet dictatorship. In a prose style that grabs its readers by the collar, Lemebel recounts the lives of individual locas—a derogatory Chilean term for a travesti, trans woman, or even an effeminate gay man—while also prompting questions about the relationship between the words we use and the way we see the world.

Throughout his work, Lemebel remains unabashedly political. He hated the word *gay*, a term he associates with the moneyed, white, and hypermasculine homosexual culture that has steamrolled homespun Latin American homosexualities, which to his mind are poor, Indigenous, and feminine. But, beyond his militant stance, what perhaps most risks getting lost in translation is Lemebel's simultaneous acridity and tenderness, a generosity toward language and the world even amid steely resistance to its conditions. His dissatisfaction with the available vocabulary is coextensive with his love for language, as his capricious conjunctions of syllables and sly wordplay become the very nodes of his resistance.

Lemebel was born in 1952, as Pedro Mardones, on the poorer outskirts of Santiago. In the crónica "Zanjón upon the Water," named for the neighborhood where he grew up, he describes his early years with irony, nostalgia, and a bit of fairy-tale dust, braiding his childhood memories of poverty with early subversive experiences of gender: after sipping, as a toddler, on the sewage that runs in the stream behind the family's home, he becomes "pregnant" with what's assumed to be a stomach virus but later turns out to be a tadpole. Even memories of his mother's physical affection feel inextricable from economic realities: his mother's hands—an image he will return to in "Manifesto" and "Street Corners of My Heart"—are "gashed by bleach."

Lemebel came of age in the seventies, studying carpentry and metallurgy at a technical school before enrolling as an art student at the University of Chile. The late 1960s had brought a blossoming of Chilean art and music, particularly the political folk music genre known as Nueva Canción (New Song)—a movement that included figures like Violeta Parra and Víctor Jara, two singer-composers that Lemebel particularly admired and whom he references in various crónicas. The Socialist leader Salvador Allende was elected president in 1970, inaugurating a period of remarkable—even utopian—political energy and hope. Allende moved to significantly increase government services, building public hospitals and housing, raising the minimum wage, creating literary and education programs, and guaranteeing free access to milk for women with children. In moves that greatly upset the wealthy Chilean establishment, he nationalized the banks and copper industry, and expanded a land seizure and redistribution program that had begun under Eduardo Frei, his Christian Democrat predecessor; by the beginning of 1973, the majority of the enormous agricultural estates had been reduced to two hundred acres.

But what began as a bright new decade turned into a tumultuous and ultimately bloody one for the country. Class tensions ran high as Allende began to enact his reforms. Following the March 1973 congressional elections, the streets were filled almost daily with marches from every side of the political spectrum—from conservative wives who protested the government's food rationing, to groups further to the left than Allende such as the Movimiento de Izquierda Revolucionaria (Revolutionary Left Movement), which wanted civilian armed resistance to counter the military's increasing distance from the presidency. The country's difficulties, which included inflation and a shrinking economy, were intensified by and in some cases created through secret US involvement—the food shortage, for example, was caused by a months-long strike by the truck drivers union, where the drivers were paid wages by the CIA in order to remain on strike indefinitely.

In June, the right-wing paramilitary group Frente Nacionalista Patria y Libertad (Fatherland and Liberty Nationalist Front) staged a failed coup; by August, the police and military commanders who supported Allende had either been forced to resign or been assassinated. And on September 11, 1973, the military, backed by the United States, staged a successful coup, bombing the presidential palace with Allende inside. During the weeks and years that followed, thousands would be detained and killed—collectively known as "the disappeared," as most of the bodies were never recovered, nor their deaths confirmed. The state was now run by a military junta—a group of four generals, with General Augusto Pinochet as head of state. The new regime implemented a nightly curfew that it maintained until 1987, shortly before Pinochet stepped down from power.

It is onto this grim stage, in the eighties, that Lemebel first steps. Not as a writer—though he has, importantly, begun attending workshops with writers Diamela Eltit and Pía Barros.

Like many Allende supporters, he spent the second half of the seventies keeping a low profile. But during the final years of the dictatorship, having been fired from his job as an art teacher for his homosexuality, he began making, together with the artist Francisco Casas, what are now considered key early pieces of Latin American performance art.

There wasn't really a word, at least not in Chile, for what they were doing back then: putting their bodies on the line in sometimes playful, at other times profoundly dangerous, situations. Calling themselves Las Yeguas del Apocalipsis ("The Mares of the Apocalypse"), the pair often appeared in drag, and their performances—equal parts brilliant and disruptive—confronted not only the dictatorship's atrocities, but also the Left's homophobia and its blindness to the rapidly developing AIDS crisis. As one of their first acts, at the ceremony where Raúl Zurita accepted the 1988 Pablo Neruda Award for Poetry, the pair climbed onstage and crowned the poet with thorns—a wink at Zurita's public gestures of self-sacrifice. In another instance, the two of them rode naked on a white horse into the campus of the University of Chile. Perhaps their most famous piece is *The Conquest of America* (1989), a bloody homosexual pas de deux in which, bare-chested and barefoot, they performed the cueca, a traditional (and often politicized) dance in Chile, over a map of South America made of glass shards from Coke bottles. This was in front of the Chilean Commission on Human Rights, the committee responsible for calculating the number of people who were killed or tortured by the Chilean military between 1973 and 1989.

Lemebel recounts some of these art actions in the crónicas. In "The Death of Madonna," he describes how, in November 1989, coinciding with one of the resistance's citywide blackouts, the Yeguas drew glowing stars on the ground, creating a Hollywood-style walk of fame and setting up a faux film premiere, which included spotlights and press coverage, so the locas in the surrounding neighborhood could pretend to be movie stars. But the action's title, *Gone with AIDS*—a twist on *Gone with the Wind*—suggests that most of those who participated would be subject to a very different fate. Lemebel's first book of crónicas, *La esquina es mi corazón* (Street corners of my heart), was published in 1995—a chapbook of short stories, *Incontables* (Uncountables) was published earlier, in 1986—and with it, Lemebel sprang into the literary world fully formed as a writer. His second book, *Loco afán* (Wild desire, 1996), brought him international attention. For it is in *Loco afán* that Lemebel places the AIDS crisis and the locas front and center, memorializing his friends who have "disappeared" in what feels to him like political déjà vu.

If we were to take Lemebel's flamboyantly baroque crónicas literally, AIDS arrived with the blond, macho gay tourist, who sank his contagious teeth into the streetwalking locas who slept with foreign men for a living. Though Lemebel often narrates the deaths of real individuals, the crónica as a form is expansive enough for him to imbue the act of dying with camp sensibility, and he casts each loca, as she falls sick, in the starring role of her own private tragedy. The distraught girls who remain behind become the chorus, eager to fulfill the elaborate last wishes of their friends. An emaciated queen's desire to star in a film, or eat tangerine ice cream, is both high-camp absurdist and entirely realistic as a portrayal of dementia, a late-stage complication of AIDS. This double vision—of being both mannered and natural, self-conscious and sincere—is a hallmark of camp, and a holdover from the years Lemebel spent performing. How can anyone be natural when being watched? The question applies equally to actors, to queers, to anyone living under surveillance. Lemebel writes like he's facing a crowd, or the firing squad. His affectation is also an urgency.

Lemebel's overwrought sentences almost succeed in distracting us, the readers, from the precarious lives of these characters, and part of his brilliance lies in his ability to depict the drama and humor of that disparity. In "The Million Names of María Chameleon," he argues for the importance of nicknames among the locas, especially for those who get sick. He follows his defense with a long list of names, filled with winks at pop culture and sexual preferences. The list becomes an homage with a dramatic arc, a compilation of symptoms that doubles as an essay on the uses of humor in crisis and resistance. But as the list progresses, so does the disease. And in the end, while there are nicknames for the dying, there are none for the dead.

Camp (or what I'm approximating as camp) also informs how Lemebel writes about the dictatorship. He often looks through the eyes of the women involved, finding a strange, cruel sympathy even with those who hew close to power, such as the wives of military generals who organize a jewelry drive for rebuilding the country, only to find their jewels on the necks of the wives of American diplomats; or the woman whose cocktail parties attract the literary elite to her living room while her husband tortures suspected dissidents in the basement. (Lemebel related this horrific scene to Roberto Bolaño, who turned it into the central premise of *By Night in Chile*.) But his tone turns serious when he recounts interviews with women who were detained by the regime, or who search for their disappeared husbands. And though his descriptions are never entirely free of irony, Lemebel touches in several crónicas on the dictatorship's end: the Left's remarkable NO campaign during the 1988 referendum on whether Pinochet should remain in power, its electoral victory the final nail in the dictatorship's coffin.

Immediately following the coup, many artists and activists had sought asylum in other countries, generating a further split between those who left and those who stayed. Perhaps this is why when Roberto Bolaño, exile par excellence to the rest of the world, returned to Chile for the first time in 1995, he expressed a certain nervousness about meeting Lemebel. But Bolaño soon became one of Lemebel's biggest supporters, and arranged to have the crónicas—which would eventually total seven slim volumes—published in Spain. (As Bolaño wryly noted, "Lemebel doesn't have to write poetry to be the best poet of my generation.") The books were lauded by the Mexican writer Carlos Monsiváis and quickly gained a readership on both sides of the Atlantic. Lemebel would go on to receive Germany's Anna Seghers Prize, the José Donoso Prize in Latin American Letters, and a Guggenheim Fellowship, with his work being translated by the early 2000s into German, French, Italian, and English, most significantly his only novel, *Tengo miedo torero*, translated by Katherine Silver as *My Tender Matador*.

By the end of his life, Lemebel would be both a popular hero and a darling—or maybe enfant terrible—of the Latin American art and literary world; a queer icon as well as an activist; someone who was constantly stopped on the street by his fans. According to one of his friends, the critic Soledad Bianchi, these fans were often women and often on the older side—an unusual readership for his unflinching stories about travesti lives. One of the first things that drew me to Lemebel was that everyone—from the twentysomething-year-old punks in the port city Valparaíso, to the highbrow literati in Santiago, to the working-class grandmothers in the provinces—seemed to have read and loved him. How could a single writer resonate with such a wide range of people?

Lemebel had reached these audiences in part because he'd expanded the kinds of media he was using to tell his stories. After publishing *La esquina es mi corazón*, he was offered a slot on Radio Tierra, a grassroots feminist station, where on his program *Cancionero* (Songbook) he read many of the crónicas that became his third collection, *De perlas y cicatrices* (Of pearls and scars). Ten or so of the original recordings of these shows remain available online; the radio felt like a particularly apt home for Lemebel, whose work is inflected with Chilean oral culture and popular music. Additionally, Lemebel began publishing pieces in newspapers and magazines with national distribution (*La Nación*, *The Clinic*, *Punto Final*, *Página Abierta*).

The shorter publication cycles for radio pieces and newspaper columns both streamlined Lemebel's style and led him to comment with more frequency on current politics. He questioned the new democratic government's protection of the old military junta under a process that was being called the "transition to democracy." Just across the cordillera of the Andes, five leaders of the Argentine military dictatorship had been successfully prosecuted in 1985 and put in jail. Pinochet, by contrast, was made a lifelong senator; eventual prosecution attempts, which began a decade later, and in Europe rather than Chile, were held up by a continual back-and-forth about impunity granted for medical reasons or political status. He died without ever having been convicted of a crime. Lemebel also objected, along with many others, to the continued use of Pinochet-era laws and the Pinochet-era constitution—especially the many free-market economic policies that the dictatorship had imported wholesale from Milton Friedman's Chicago seminars. He voiced a growing suspicion among much of the public that nothing, or not nearly enough, had changed, especially in the face of the country's extreme economic inequality.

When Lemebel died in early 2015, of laryngeal cancer, hundreds attended his boisterous, celebratory wake, filled with music and dancing; and the government threw him an equally lavish, now legendary funeral, where Chile's luminaries and locas all gathered to say their goodbyes. Upon hearing of Lemebel's death, the novelist Alejandro Zambra wrote that his work "is studied all over, he is talked about in the press, on the radio, on TV, because his books created an audience that didn't exist before. His books changed lives. To say that his work is important for Chilean literature would be stingy: his work is important for Chile." And four years later, in October 2019, when protests exploded in the streets over a thirty-peso subway fare hike that became a flash point for deeper grievances (with thousands shouting, "It's not thirty pesos, it's thirty years!"), a social movement eventually resulting in a national plebiscite that voted out the Pinochet-era constitution, Lemebel's face was everywhere, painted on murals and signs and barricades.

I am often asked whether Lemebel would be considered trans in our contemporary understanding, and his characters trans women. I began translating Lemebel's work in 2016, and finished in 2023. In those intervening years, the public conversation around gender identity in the US and the UK has changed significantly, as has the conversation in Latin America. The travestis and locas in the crónicas, though far too often fated to live lives cut short, are also marked by a sense of uncontainability. For Lemebel, loca identity was something simultaneously uncompromising and malleable: he intentionally used terms and pronouns quite loosely, valuing playfulness, possibility, and a notion of desborde (literally meaning overflow or excess).

And I am pulled, as a translator always is, between writer and eager reader, between building bridges and holding the line. On the one hand, I need to honor Lemebel's cultural and temporal specificities—he never identified as trans—and respect his broader, explicit refusal of the Global North's gender and sexuality identifiers, which he saw as a colonial imposition. It's hard to describe in contemporary English, replete with specific identifiers that can imply a high level of access to medical care, the expansiveness of the travesti identity in Spanish and its disassociation from hormone therapy or surgeries, especially in the 1980s and '90s. Many if not most travestis still make their living as sex workers, and certainly did back then. As the scholar Melissa M. González points out in the *Postposttransexual* issue of *Transgender Studies Quarterly*, Lemebel saw locas as historically and culturally specific, destined to disappear with globalized capitalism. On the other hand, many today in Latin America identify both as trans and as a loca. Perhaps importantly, too, I find myself peering into a yawning gap that is the lack of a trans canon in our collective literary imagination.

Once, cooking lunch with a Chilean American friend, a talented younger writer at the early stages of exploring their gender identity, I pressed the point that Lemebel was not, in fact, trans. Their face fell. Years later, my friend is out as trans, cheerfully insisting over an international phone call that Lemebel definitely wouldn't have called himself trans and describing the ongoing debate around Lemebel's pronouns in Chile. So we're on the same page, and yet—I still remember her face falling. The strength of that memory has made me wonder: What am I accomplishing by gatekeeping? Who is Lemebel writing for, if not for her?

A trans canon sounds like an oxymoron; I don't know whether Lemebel would be horrified or gleeful to have infiltrated Penguin Classics (possibly a little of both). He wrote urgently, for his own time, his own friends, and yet his rollicking quicksilver sentences are built to last. He's a cult classic—meaning a classic in a skewed, through-the-back-door kind of way, in a passed-from-hand-to-hand, mouth-to-mouth, slid-over-bar-countertops, or dropped-in-a-mailbox kind of way. What I love most about cult classics is that there's room for everything—for cliché and for camp and for bad taste. There's room for you and room for me and room for whoever comes next. This last point mattered very much to Lemebel. So to close, here is Pedro in "Manifesto"; he is speaking, during the dictatorship, in heels, at a resistance meeting:

> So that the revolution does not completely rot
> I leave you with a message
> Not for my sake
> I am old
> And your utopia is for future generations
> There are so many children who will be born
> With a little broken wing
> And I want them to fly, comrade
> I want your revolution
> To drop them a piece of red heaven
> So that they fly.

A LAST THOUGHT ON AIDS

A good friend of mine died while I was translating this book. Her name was Cecilia Paz Peralta, and I miss her very much. She died from cancer, not from AIDS, but in helping care for her, in watching the healthcare system in Chile fail so dramatically that it became partially responsible for her death, and in clashing, sometimes bitterly, over her resulting desperate pursuit of unproven treatments, ranging from kambo to crystals to psychotherapy, I gained a tiny, limited window into certain aspects of the AIDS crisis in the 1980s and '90s, and was reminded of what many of Lemebel's crónicas are really about.

Throughout the crónicas, Lemebel refers to the disease simply as AIDS, rather than HIV or HIV/AIDS, as is now standard in the United States. Little was known then about the disease (Lemebel often calls it *the shadow* or *the mystery*), and death came quickly to those who contracted it. Even after the discovery of life-saving drugs—a result of ACT UP activists in the US demanding research and clinical trials—these prescriptions remained largely unavailable to poor locas in Chile. And today, though advancements in treatment and prevention mean that HIV is now a manageable disease, 650,000 people worldwide die annually from AIDS-related causes. Meanwhile, in the US, HIV/AIDS continues to disproportionately affect communities of color, and 30,000 people receive positive diagnoses each year. It is remarkable and damning how little we talk or think about it as a larger culture.

Still, the AIDS crisis—i.e., the period of time before there was any known medical treatment—registers very differently for those who remember it and those who don't. The hope, from everyone involved in putting this book together, is that Lemebel's work will speak to both generations of readers. In his *New Yorker* essay about a revival of *Angels in America*, the writer and critic Hilton Als laments how younger generations, "too young to know how AIDS decimated not only a community but the world," subsequently "can't understand the love and the urgency that the play grew out of." At the same time, he questions the "maddening" vision of race and sexual difference that Tony Kushner's play presents. Lemebel's crónicas seem to answer the implicit call, helping us all remember the AIDS crisis with renewed generosity and rage.

GWENDOLYN HARPER

Suggestions for Further Reading

Lemebel's full bibliography in Spanish is as follows:

Incontables (1986 chapbook; republished Santiago: Seix Barral, 2018)

La esquina es mi corazón. Crónica urbana (Santiago: Cuarto Propio, 1995)

Loco afán. Crónicas de sidario (Santiago: LOM, 1996)

De perlas y cicatrices. Crónicas radiales (Santiago: LOM, 1998)

Tengo miedo torero (Santiago: Seix Barral, 2001)

Zanjón de la Aguada (Santiago: Seix Barral, 2003)

Adiós mariquita linda (Santiago: Sudamericana, 2004)

Serenata cafiola (Santiago: Seix Barral, 2008)

Háblame de amores (Santiago: Seix Barral, 2012)

Poco hombre. Crónicas escogidas (Santiago: Ediciones Universidad Diego Portales, 2013)

Mi amiga Gladys (Santiago: Seix Barral, 2016)

In English:

My Tender Matador, translated by Katherine Silver (New York: Grove Press, 2003)

You can also watch the recent Spanish-language film adaption of *My Tender Matador*, *Tengo miedo torero* (2020), directed by Rodrigo Sepúlveda and starring Alfredo Castro. A documentary on Lemebel's life, *Lemebel* (2019), by Joanna Reposi Garibaldi, is also available and features footage of Lemebel from both his early performance years and his final months of life.

Gloria Camiruaga's 1990 documentary *Casa particular* (available both online and in the archives of the Museo de la Memoria y los Derechos Humanos in Santiago) includes glimpses of both Lemebel and Francisco Casas as Las Yeguas del Apocalipsis, as well as certain elements that show up in crónicas like "Night of Furs" and "The Death of Madonna"; the crónica "Act Like Nothing Happened, Dream It Never Could" is a response to Camiruaga's 2000 film *La venda* (The blindfold).

For even more visual context, Paz Errázuriz's series of photographs *La manzana de Adán* (Adam's apple) documents travesti life in both Santiago and Talca in the 1980s. For a deeper look at the intersection of AIDS and literature specifically, see Lina Meruane's *Viral Voyages: Tracing AIDS in Latin America* (trans. Andrea Rosenberg; New York: Palgrave Macmillan, 2014).

A number of writers have published essays about the importance of Lemebel's work and their personal encounters with him; a few are in English or have recently been translated as part of larger essay collections. Garth Greenwell's homage to the writer was published in *The New Yorker* shortly after Lemebel's death. Roberto Bolaño's meditations on Lemebel can be found in *Between Parentheses* (ed. Ignacio Echevarría and trans. Natasha Wimmer; New York: New Directions, 2011). Two essays about Lemebel by Alejandro Zambra are included in Zambra's collection *Not to Read* (trans. Megan McDowell; London: Fitzcarraldo, 2018). Lemebel also makes a memorable cameo in Paul B. Preciado's *Testo Junkie* (first published as Beatriz Preciado; trans. Bruce Benderson; New York: Feminist Press, 2013).

For readers of Spanish, Óscar Contardo's *Loca fuerte* (Santiago: Ediciones Universidad Diego Portales, 2022) and Soledad Bianchi's *Lemebel* (Santiago: Montacerdos, 2018) are full of insights about the writer. And you can hear from Lemebel himself in *Lemebel oral. 20 años de entrevistas* (ed. Gonzalo León; Buenos Aires: Mansalva, 2018).

A Note on the Translation

This book can be read cover to cover or cruised piece to piece. I've divided the crónicas thematically, though Lemebel's intersectional subjects inevitably permeate and contaminate each other. The first section introduces us to Lemebel's queer subject matter and idiosyncratic style; the second focuses on the coup and the years of dictatorship; the third covers the AIDS crisis and contains some of Lemebel's most memorable crónicas. The fourth shifts the focus back to national politics and life in Chile after the dictatorship ended in December 1989—the neutrality of the section title, "Post-90," comes from Lemebel's refusal to use any of the new government's self-congratulatory language about the period. And the final section features crónicas that describe Lemebel's childhood and urban life in Santiago, as well as his musings about language, colonialism, and Indigeneity.

The Spanish-language volume *Poco hombre*, selected and edited by Ignacio Echevarría in consultation with Lemebel, spans Lemebel's entire writing career and served as the jumping-off point for this volume; about two thirds of our selection overlaps with that book. We placed a perhaps stronger emphasis on Lemebel's first two collections of crónicas—*La esquina es mi corazón* and *Loco afán*—while not including some pieces that didn't successfully translate beyond the specificities of Chilean culture and politics.

In truth, all of Lemebel's crónicas have been described, rightly or wrongly, as untranslatable. The split between writer and reader—between two languages, cultures, and eras—is the oldest, most basic question of international literature. As a translator, I owe the writer as close a correspondence as possible to the vision of the work (sentence for sentence, even sound for sound), just as I owe the reader access to that vision. Should I put the reader at ease, potentially compromising the more foreign or undigestible aspects of the work, or should I push the reader's willingness to read strange English and hear unfamiliar terms?

At the start of the introduction, I quoted a line from Lemebel about refusing to "kowtow" to English. I like my choice of *kowtow*, by the way: the word in Spanish is *arrodillado*, kneeling, which I could have used in the translation easily enough. But *kowtow*, from the Cantonese *kautau* (literally knock-head, to touch one's head to the ground as a sign of deep respect), seemed so much more apt, the word itself a vestige of the West's colonial encounters with imperial China in the nineteenth century. And though the word slips into English disdainfully—indicating obsequiousness rather than respect—I can't help thinking that Lemebel would relish the linguistic subterfuge and, were he writing in English, wouldn't be able to pass up the irony in this particular sentence, the Cantonese word resisting and muddying the waters even as the world's languages are forced to bow before globalizing, colonial English.

Were he writing in English. That's often used as a gloss, in translation, for loyalty to the reader and "target language." In contrast, siding with the original sounds purer, worthier, more uncompromising, especially in a world such as ours, where globalization, as Lemebel points out, has rendered so much so similar. But Lemebel, in those two sentences above, is not so much talking about English translation per se as he is talking about Spanishes—condemning the loss of rich provincial heterogeneity and the many writers who contribute to the shared illusion of a neutral, educated Spanish, often with an eye to being translated for a global market. Lemebel, by contrast, scrapes the bottom-feeder murk of Chilean slang and idioms, things that sound, to a "neutral" Spanish ear, alternately vulgar, hokey, throwback, and coded. He deals in linguistic tongue-in-cheek and the occasional triple pun. In opposition to the cultivated neutrality of the Chilean upper class and literary Spanish, Lemebel's hyper-Chilean Spanish pushes the uninitiated out. And though Lemebel was in fact hungry for artistic success, he wasn't interested in being diluted, made more palatable, or having equals signs drawn between his subject matter and "the first world."

Unsurprisingly, throughout the translation process, *travesti* and *loca* seemed to need to remain as particular identities and terms. *Travesti* can arguably be translated as *trannie*: part of the logic for keeping *travesti* was just how visually similar the two words are, the text helping build a linguistic and cultural bridge between the two terms while honoring the wholeness and irreducibility of each. And I thought *loca* especially deserved to enter the English reader's lexicon—Idra Novey, in a conversation we had shortly before I wrote this note, pointed out the way the word *loca*, repeated again and again, accrues almost the quality of an incantation in Lemebel's work. My hope is that the translation manages to re-create this summoning to life.

The book *Gay New York: Gender, Urban Culture, and the Making of the Gay Male World, 1890–1940*, by George Chauncey, showed me a version of historical queer life in the United States that had useful, surprisingly close analogies to the world Lemebel describes; there was also significant, serendipitous metaphorical overlap, which gave me some amount of direction and confidence when translating. I ultimately translated the Chilean pejorative slang word *cola*—which means an animal's tail, or a queue, or someone's butt, or a loca—as *fairy*, *pansy*, or occasionally *sissy*. Halfway between a slur and an endearment, the word *cola* exemplifies Lemebel's loving, explicit reappropriation of derogatory language. He stuffs his crónicas with jokes and imaginative variants on this word (*coliza*, *colita*, *colipato*, *coliflor*, *coliguacho*) and I let context guide my translations in some cases, depending on whatever made the most sense for the larger image or puns at play and for the syntactic rhythm. Other terms fell into place more easily: *homosexual* was *homosexual*; *maricón* more or less equals *fag* or *faggot*. And *reina* obviously translates into *queen*—though when Lemebel uses the word, he means to connote a queen bee or loca who's calling the social shots.

Translator's Acknowledgments

Lemebel's work is experiencing a revival—his novel and crónicas have recently been translated into languages as diverse as Arabic, Croatian, Portuguese, and Thai, among many others, and his work is being reissued in Spain. None of this would be possible without the many people who have tended the Lemebel flame all these years; I'm especially grateful to Felipe Gana Gómez de la Torre at Ediciones Universidad Diego Portales for both shepherding that initial anthology of crónicas and giving his blessing for this one.

In the US, John Siciliano at Penguin Classics provided a steady hand and clear head, keeping the complex project on course throughout the process. In the UK, Rory Williamson at Pushkin Press kept my spirits up from an ocean away and offered additional invaluable support, especially with crónica selection. Thank you, too, to the many people behind the scenes at each of these presses, who cared for this book down to the last detail: Elda Rotor, Marissa Davis, Elizabeth Pham Janowski, Pedro Martin, Katie Hurley, Elizabeth Yaffe, and Julia Rickard at Penguin, and Adam Freudenheim, Jo Walker, and Steven Cooper at Pushkin.

The agent Elianna Kan made miracles happen through her passion and dedication to Lemebel's work. Paz Errázuriz, renowned photographer and longtime friend of Lemebel's, generously provided the image for both the US and UK covers. Additional thanks go to Daniela Mardones Caro and the entire Lemebel family for entrusting the editors and myself with this important work, and to Josefina Alemparte Balmaceda at Planeta for facilitating the rights. Emily Wolahan and George

Henson, editors at *Two Lines* and *Latin American Literature Today*, respectively, published early versions of several crónicas. The National Endowment for the Arts and the Robert B. Silvers Foundation awarded translation grants for the project at key moments that enabled me to continue working on the manuscript.

A number of people nudged this project along less formally by encouraging, reading pages, or discussing it with me: Esther Allen, Austin Carder, Elias Chen, Mónica de la Torre, Katrina Dodson, Garth Greenwell, Lina Meruane, Idra Novey, Nico Vela Page, Aldo Perán, Julia Powers, Katherine Silver, Stephanie Wong, Alice Yang, and the Bay Area Literary Translators' Working Group. I'm particularly grateful to friends in Chile and Argentina, especially Carmín Rodríguez and Sofía Böhmer. Thank you to my family, real and fake, and to Govind. And, finally, this translation would not exist at all without two people: Peter Cole, who taught me to translate and who continues to be generous with his time and thoughts, and Sergio Parra, who took me seriously when, as a stammering stranger, I walked into his bookshop and told him that I'd like to translate Leme[illegible]ank you both.

Chronology

1952 Pedro Mardones Lemebel born in Santiago, Chile.

1964 Eduardo Frei elected president as a Christian Democrat.

1969 First Festival of Chilean Nueva Canción held in Santiago.

The vast majority of leftist political parties in Chile formally band together under a new coalition, Popular Unity.

1970 Salvador Allende, longtime senator and former health minister, elected president as the Popular Unity candidate.

1973 Allende deposed in a US-backed military coup on September 11. Augusto Pinochet appointed head of the military junta, a group of four generals who jointly govern Chile for the next seven years. DINA (National Intelligence Directorate) established.

1974 General Carlos Prats, Allende loyalist, assassinated while in voluntary exile in Buenos Aires.

1975 Operation Condor formalized as a transnational cooperation among secret police in military dictatorships across the Southern Cone, particularly Chile and Argentina but extending to Brazil, Uruguay, Bolivia, and Paraguay, and further assisted by US military and intelligence.

1976 Orlando Letelier, a political exile, assassinated in Washington, DC.

1977 DINA dissolved, replaced by the CNI (National Information Center).

1980 A new constitution is approved by a potentially rigged plebiscite; with it, the military junta is dissolved and Pinochet is appointed president for an eight-year term.

1981 *The New York Times* publishes an article with the headline, "Rare Cancer Seen in 41 Homosexuals."

1984 First recorded cases of HIV/AIDS in Chile.

1986 Lemebel reads "Manifesto" at a leftist resistance meeting against the dictatorship. Publishes chapbook *Incontables.*

1987 Lemebel and Francisco Casas form Las Yeguas del Apocalipsis.

ACT UP, the AIDS Coalition to Unleash Power, is formed in New York City.

1988 A second national plebiscite is held in Chile, over whether Pinochet can remain in power another eight years or must step down and hold democratic elections. The NO campaign wins the vote that results in ousting Pinochet.

1989 Las Yeguas perform *The Conquest of America* for the Chilean Commission on Human Rights.

Patricio Aylwin elected to the presidency, forms National Commission for Truth and Reconciliation.

1991 The National Commission for Truth and Reconciliation Report, also known as the Rettig Report, is released, with the names of more than two thousand individuals killed or disappeared during the dictatorship (the majority between 1973 and 1977).

1994 Lemebel participates in the twenty-fifth anniversary of the Stonewall riots in New York.

1995 *La esquina es mi corazón* published.

1996 *Loco afán* published. Lemebel begins broadcasting episodes of *Cancionero*, a ten-minute program on Radio Tierra where he reads his crónicas.

1996 Two new drugs, Crixivan and Norvir, when taken in combination with the already available AZT or ddI, are shown to be effective at extended suppression of the HIV virus; they soon become available in the US, meaningfully changing the course of HIV/AIDS for most patients.

1998 *De perlas y cicatrices* published.

Elimination of national holiday celebrating the military coup. Pinochet arrested in his hospital room at The London Clinic by British special agents for human rights violations.

The Clinic, a satirical progressive newspaper, is founded in Chile and begins publishing Lemebel's crónicas as a regular column.

1999 *Loco afán* published in Spain. Lemebel attends Guadalajara Book Fair and receives Guggenheim Fellowship. Homosexuality legalized in Chile.

2000 Longtime resistance leader Ricardo Lagos elected president. After sixteen months of house arrest in London, Pinochet sent back to Chile and declared immune from prosecution due to medical issues. The "Mesa de Diálogo" (Table for Dialogue) is held between religious leaders, the military, and several members of civil society.

2001 *Tengo miedo torero* (*My Tender Matador*) published.

2003 *Zanjón de la Aguada* ("Zanjón upon the Water") published.

2004 *Adiós mariquita linda* published.

2006 Lemebel receives Anna Seghers Prize.

2008 *Serenata cafiola* published.

2012 *Háblame de amores* published.

2013 *Poco hombre*, a selection of Lemebel's crónicas, published in Chile. Lemebel receives José Donoso Prize.

2015 Lemebel dies from laryngeal cancer on January 23.

2016 *Mi amiga Gladys* published.

2019 The "30 pesos" social revolution. *Lemebel* documentary premieres.

2020 *My Tender Matador* feature film premieres. Chilean national plebiscite votes to overturn military-era constitution and form a constitutional convention.

A Last Supper of Queer Apostles

To Olga Lemebel,
my grandmother, wayward affection and single mother.

To Violeta Lemebel,
the woman who gave me voice.

To Carmen Berenguer,
for the friendship of her pen's wild feather.

To Francisco Casas,
for the Yeguas del Apocalipsis and the traces of that ashy carnival.

To Polo Escárate,
whom we called La Pola Negri.

To Elías Jamet,
who lived on Calle Paris.

To Néstor Perlongher,
we met up in Valparaíso, the last time.

To Juan Edmundo González,
I said goodbye to him window-shopping on Paseo Ahumada.

To Sigifredo Barra,
I remember your hat with its leopard-print ribbon.

To holy luck.

To dangerous passion.

To so many.

The plague arrived like a new way of
colonizing, through a virus.

It turned our feathers into syringes, and
the sun into a frozen drop of moon through the
window.

IN LIEU OF A SYNOPSIS

I could write neat and clear, without so many nooks and crannies, so much useless pinwheeling. I could write almost telegraphically for the whole world and for the symmetrical ratification of all languages kowtowed to English. I'll never write in English; with any luck I say, *Go home*. I could write a doorstopper of a novel with weighty silences and an elaborate plot; I could write the silence of the Dao with its fastidiousness for the precise word, while stuffing my adjectives under a disciplined tongue. I could write with no tongue, like a newscaster on CNN, no accent and hold the salt. But my tongue is salted and the syllables, rather than correcting me, they sing. I could write to correct, to pass on knowledge, so that my mess of a tongue might learn to sit down and be quiet. I could write with my legs crossed and buttocks tight, with Sufi yearning and the Orient's economy of language. I could improve my language, shoving every last corroded metaphor up my ass, along with my stinking desires and hysterical mind full of Mary Lou or Marry AIDS, with no parasol or with my umbrella propped upside down, right in the sun so that I go global, exportable, translated even into Greek, which sings to me about as much as a blossoming fart. I could hide away the ire and plumed rage of my images, the violence enacted by violence, and sleep peacefully with my romantic fantasies. But that's not who I am—I concocted my name with the milonga drag of a travestango starlet, a faggy cueca or hard rock bolero. I could report on the high life and come to regret my coarse and lurid subject matter. Leave the rabble-rousing to the rabble and dig through Hispanic etymology instead. But that's not why I came. The world is full of writers with fountain pens staining flowers into the miserly buttonholes of their lapels. I didn't come to sing *ladies and gentlemen*; but all the same I do sing, my dear señora. I don't know why I showed up at this concert, but here I am. And the verses flew from me like a knife. But not really verses, just my hand drawing out the growl, the sob. Like the screech of a cowardly bitch, certain writers hissed from the right wing of the stage. I came to writing with no love for it, I was heading somewhere else, I wanted to sing protest songs, fly on the trapeze, or be an Indian bird trilling at the dusk. But my tongue curled up in impotence and instead of clarity or studied emotion I emitted a jungle of sounds. I wasn't musical, I wasn't singing within earshot of higher powers so they'd remember me at the right hand of neoliberal heaven. My father wondered why they paid me to write while nobody rewarded him for the effort. And I did learn by effort, I learned already grown, just like Paquita la del Barrio. Writing didn't come easy to me. I wanted to sing and they clubbed me with rules. I learned clawing my way through onomatopoeia, dieresis, intonation, and the big knockers of grammar and spelling. But so many rules were bad for me, so many crosswords of thought, and I forgot it all instantly. I learned out of hunger, out of necessity, from working at it, from pimping myself, but I began to feel sad. I could've written like the others and in a style that was beautiful and clear, as clear as the water that runs through Patagonia's rivers. But the city did me wrong, mistreated me, and sex drew its X and spat on my sphincter. I say that I could, but really I couldn't have—I lacked rigor, and getting fucked up won out, the sordid charm of love lied. And like an idiot I believed, like a drooping skank I hoodwinked with baroque allegories and nonsense that sounded real nice. You could've been someone else, the teachers told me, drool staining their haircloths. Despite everything I did learn, but sadness fell on me like a cloak. I said I wasn't a singer and that's true, but music was the only technicolor in my tipsy biography. And here's the staff where the story lurches out its tragic rhythms. Like it or not, I'll press play on this last collection of songs.

MARICÓN

HER THROATY LAUGH
(OR, THE TRAVESTI STREETWALKER'S SWEET DECEIT)

The travesti who walks the streets is the wonder of the witching hour, a flash of mother-of-pearl catching the light in a city whorehouse hallway. Just a fairytail wink, a fluttering of lashes, a baring of implants under the bright traffic lights bloodying the street corner where the sharp work of a whore's soul clicks its heels.

In the pouring rain, teeth chattering, warming the wait with a bummed cigarette: her nightly travesti tango is a quick glance, a chance wink that unnerves, that at first convinces the passerby but whose jaw then goes slack, eyes glued to the sheen at her neckline skating down the cleavage of sexual deception. But the tug of this streetwalking masquerade is never all that innocent, since playing the game is what seduces most men, who always know, who always suspect that this platinum bombshell is not so womanly after all. Something in her exaggerated staging goes too far. Something runneth over in her girlish, throaty laugh. She overtakes the feminine in her six feet, plus heels. She hams it up with her pursed lips asking for a smoke from the shadows. The future client knows what plastered makeup means, its geisha theater, but he lets his own deceit draw him in, fastening his desire to the nylon wings of those down-and-out fairies who circle the city's roundabouts. Those night herons whose long legs extend far past Coco Chanel and her demure miniskirts. The bewitched future lover prefers not to think about what's hiding below that rag, a surprise, a DIY slipknot surgery, where transsexuality is its own law, its own traffic, detouring a husband who was on his way home. The stressed office worker in a car he bought on credit, who doesn't want to get back just to watch *¿Cuánto vale el show?*, who hates returning early and having to listen to his wife serve a platter of complaints and regrets and unpaid bills. So he stops the car to toss in a drifting glamorous apparition, that insect clinging to the rearview mirror who in a single jump makes herself at home in the passenger seat. And after the high-wire pirouettes of a wholesale haggle, they reach an agreement and clinch the deal by nixing the motel cost in favor of the Toyota's reclinable seat.

Afterward, the travesti returns to her outpost in the urban jungle, counting the money from her quickie session. Subtracting the handful of bills from a Chilean family's monthly costs, there's still not enough to pay rent, never mind buy those Cinderella slippers that she saw downtown. Not nearly enough for her mother and younger siblings, who cost more than a night out with Claudia Schiffer. Her poor mama, the only one who understands her, who fixes her wig and tucks condoms into her purse, telling her to be careful, that men are bad and how she should never get into a car with more than one of them, how she should write the license plate down just in case they leave her tits up and covered with cigarette burns, like what happened to poor Wendy last week. How she's too worried to sleep, praying that la Virgen will keep her little girl safe from the night's dangers. But the loca just shrugs, saying work is like that, she never knows if tomorrow, in some corner of Santiago, her migratory flights might end in a ditch. She never knows if a stray bullet or police raid, like Death's stork, will cut short her breath. Maybe this very Friday night, when there are so many clients, when teenagers from uptown chuck bottles at her for fun as they drive by. When her high heel breaks right as she's running to meet a yellow Lada and La Susi beats her to it, La Susi, who's younger than her and who always wins. This could be the last time she sees the city emerge from dawn's pink cotton sheets. And she's so alone, so numb, so sparrowlike with her belly full of dreams, exposed to daylight's morality as the sun rises and slashes her work's sweet deceit.

MANIFESTO

(I SPEAK FROM MY DIFFERENCE)

I am not Pasolini asking for explanations
I am not Ginsberg thrown out of Cuba
I am not a faggot masking as a poet
I need no mask
Here is my face
I speak from my difference
Defend what I am
I am not so strange
I smell injustice
And mistrust this democratic cueca
But don't speak to me about the proletariat
Because being poor and a fag is worse
One must be acid to bear it
It's steering clear of the macho kids on the corner
It's a father who hates you
Because his son's hips swing too much
It's having a mother whose hands are gashed by bleach
Aged with cleaning
Holding you like a child grown sick
Through bad habits
Through bad luck
Like the dictatorship
Worse than the dictatorship
Because the dictatorship ends
And democracy arrives
With socialism tiptoeing behind
And then?

What will you do with us, comrade?
Will you bundle us by our braids for shipment to Cuban quarantine?
Will you stick us inside some train to nowhere
Like General Ibáñez's big boat
Where we learned how to swim
But no one ever made it to shore
And so Valparaíso turned out its red lights
And so the houses of caramba
Shed us a black tear
For the fairies consumed by crabs
That year the Commission on Human Rights can't remember
And so dear comrade I ask you
Does reactionary propaganda's train still exist, heading for Siberia?
The train that passes through your pupils
When my voice turns too sweet
And you?
What will you do with that memory of boys jerking each other off and other stuff
on holiday in Cartagena?
Will the future be in black and white?
Time strictly divided into night and working day?
Won't there be a fag on some corner upsetting the future of your New Man?
Will you let us embroider birds onto the flag of this free country?
The rifle I'll leave with you
Who has colder blood
And don't think it's fear
Fear left me
With each intercepted blade
In the bordello basements where I lived
And don't feel insulted
If I speak to you about these things
And look at your bulge
I am not a hypocrite
Perhaps a woman's tits don't make you lower your eyes?

Don't you think that alone in the mountains
    something might happen between us?
Although you'd hate me afterward
For corrupting your moral revolution
Are you scared of homosexualizing life?
I'm not talking about putting it in and pulling it out
And pulling it out and putting it in, not just that
I speak of sweetness, comrade
You have no idea
What it costs to find love
In these conditions
You have no idea
What it means to carry this leprosy
People keep their distance
People understand and say:
He's a fag but writes well
He's a fag but a friend
Super easygoing
I am not easygoing
I accept the world
Without asking that it go easy
But either way they laugh
I've got scars of laughter on my spine
You suppose I think with my tush
That with one round on the CNI's electric grill
Everything would come tumbling out
You don't know that manhood was not
Something I learned in those chambers
The night taught me manhood
Behind a post
That manhood you boast about
Was snuck into your ranks
A trained killer
Sent by those still in power
The Party didn't give me my manhood
Because they rejected me chuckling
Many times
Manhood was something I learned by sharing

In the worst of those years
And they laughed at my faggy voice
Shouting: *And they will fall, and they will fall*
And though you shout like a man
You have not managed to make them go
My manhood was biting the gag
Not going to the stadium
And throwing punches over Colo-Colo
Football is homosexuality in plain sight
Just like boxing, politics, and wine
My manhood was to swallow your taunts
To eat my rage rather than kill the whole world
My manhood is to know myself different
To be a coward is harder
I do not turn the other cheek
I turn my ass comrade
And that is my revenge
My manhood waits patiently
For the machos to grow old
Because at this stage of the game
The Left trades its droopy ass
For a seat in parliament
My manhood was difficult
And so I'm not getting on this train
Without knowing where it goes
I will not change for Marxism
Which rejected me so many times
I don't need to change
I am more subversive than you
I will not change simply
Because the poor and the rich
Have other bones to pick
Or because capitalism is unjust
In New York the fags kiss in the street
But that part I leave to you
Since you're so interested
So that the revolution does not completely rot
I leave you with a message

Not for my sake
I am old
And your utopia is for future generations
There are so many children who will be born
With a little broken wing
And I want them to fly, comrade
I want your revolution
To drop them a piece of red heaven
So that they fly.

This text was read as an intervention during a left-wing political action that occurred in September 1986 in Santiago, Chile.

ANACONDAS IN THE PARK

And despite the man-made lightning that scrapes intimacy from the parks with its halogen spies, where municipal razor blades have shaved the grass's chlorophyll into waves of plush green. Yards upon yards of *verde que te quiero verde* in Parque Forestal all straightened up, pretending to be some creole Versailles, like a scenic backdrop for democratic leisure. Or more like a terrarium, like Japanese landscaping, where even the weeds are subject to the bonsai salon's military buzzcuts. Where security cameras the mayor dreamed up now dry up the saliva of a kiss in the bigoted chemistry of urban control. Cameras so they can romanticize a beautiful park painted in oils, with blond children on swing sets, their braids flying in the wind. Lights and lenses hidden by the flower in the senator's buttonhole, so they can keep an eye on all the dementia drooling on the benches. Old-timers with watery blue eyes and poodle pooches cropped by the same hand that hacks away at the cypresses.

But even then, with all this surveillance, somewhere past the sunset turning bronze in the city smog. In the shadows that fall outside the diameter of grass recruited by the streetlamps. Barely touching the wet basting stitch of thicket, the top of a foot peeks out, then stiffens and sinks its nails into the dirt. A foot that's lost its sneaker in the straddling of rushed sex, the public space paranoia. Extremities entwine, legs arching and dry paper lips that rasp, "Not so hard, that hurts, slowly now, oh, careful, someone's coming."

Couples walk by on the path, holding hands, gathering bouquets of orange blossoms on their way down legality's shining aisle. Future newlyweds who pretend they don't see the cohabiting snakes rubbing against each other in the grass. Who say under their breath, "Those were two men, did you notice?" and keep walking, thinking about their future male children, the boys, warning them about the parks, about those types who walk alone at night and watch couples from behind the bushes. Like that voyeur who was watching them just a little while ago. He watched as they made love in the sweetness of the park because they didn't have money for a motel, but they enjoyed it more than ever, there in the green outdoors, with that spectator who couldn't applaud because his hands were busy running full steam ahead, leaking out an "Ay, I'm going to come, slow down won't you." So the woman said to the man, "You know I can't if someone's watching." But at that stage, "I can't" was a moan silenced by fever and "someone's watching" just a sprinkling of Egyptian eyes swimming among the leaves. An overwhelming vertigo that bred a pair of bronze pupils inside her, in the eyes that sprung from her pregnancy. And when the boy turned fifteen, she didn't say, "Be careful in parks," because she knew those golden eyes were the park's thirsty leaves. That's why the warning stuck in her throat. Maybe "Be careful in parks" sums up that green gossamer, that hurried drawing back of his young foreskin's curtain. That launching of himself into the park to wander over the gravel like an asp in heat, playing the fool, he smokes a cigarette so that the man following him can ask for a light and say, "What are you up to?" And, already knowing the reply, gently pushes him behind the bushes. And there, in all that damp, he kindles the curled pubic forest, his lizard tongue sucking on balls of wild hierbabuena. His fiery kiss climbing to the tip of that selenite stem. And while cars and buses careen along the ribbon of coastline, the boy hands over all the stagnation of his fragile fifteen years, years now shipwrecked like paper boats in the soaked sheets of grass. And who cares if the rustling branches tell him that someone is watching, because he knows how hard it is to see a porn movie in this country; he's watched before, too, and he's familiar with the technique, parting branches to join the park's incestuous trinity.

Maybe watching is like assisting a murder, strangling the victim's voodoo doll until it drips its rattlesnake poison down your fingers. The watched scene is repeated behind glassy irises, a carbon copy in the tear ducts, like generous handouts to satisfy the hunger of anyone watching. That's why the park's humidity melts the adolescent into an anonymous pervert. That's why each night seeps into the crisscross of his feathers and he doesn't mind coagulating with the other men, who snake along the path like lost anacondas, like cobras with jeweled hoods who recognize each other by the urgent stoplight of their rubies.

Laborers and students, office workers and seminarians—they all transform into ophidians who shed their uniforms, their dry skin, tribalizing desire in rattles of opaque becoming. Their steady gazes hold something abject enough to accumulate a Sahara, an Atacama, dusty salt-flat fields that hiss in the parched trident of their tongues. Barely a drizzle of semen fraying the lips, a silvery strand of drool shooting straight to the burrowed heart of a nest ribboned with toilet paper, which absorbs the leaking tears. Nests for a clutch of condoms that collect in the meadows like stuffed cabbage rolls of polyethylene, waiting for the sun to ferment them in the magnolias' saffron mulch.

At night the parks blossom in a dew of lonely pearls, a shower of rice that spills in the circle jerk, an ecosystem of passion that surrounds the consummating couple. Collective masturbations that recycle childhood games in their frenzied handiwork: the toboggan, the swing set, the seesaw, hide-and-go-seek in the dark with fraternities of men, rudders erect, who cling to each other as the cartilage adds up. Cock in hand, hand in hand and cock askew, they form a round that collectivizes the rejected act in a carousel of fondling, in a blindman's bluff of touches and grasps. A tribal dance where anyone can hook their caboose to the midnight express, its rails the warp for a cocoon woven in the penetrating and being penetrated beneath the swirling acacia trees. An ancestral rite in a milky ring that reflects the full moon, bouncing its light into the centrifuge of shyer voyeurs whose hearts throb in the tachycardia of brass knuckles between the weeds. Nights of ring-around-the-rosy that break off like a pearl necklace at the police's whistle, at the siren's searching purple, its blinking strobe that bloodies the party, breaking it into flashes of buttock and scrotum. At the clean thwacks striking the law into the hollow drums of their backs, to the safari rhythms of bigoted phallacies. They dodge beatings as they try to get away but fall to the ground, pants shackling them, hands covering their stunned sexual gladioli, still leafless and warm. The flashlights scour the weeds, lashing at haunches camouflaged by the cool velvet of violets. Trembling beneath the hydrangea bushes, the rookie closes the zipper biting into his pelvis—he'll change his underwear when he gets home. Someone makes a run for it by zigzagging between the cars on the highway, gunshots trailing him all the way to the bridge. In a suicidal leap, he flies over the railing and falls into the river, its waters swallowing him. The body turns up days later in Parque de los Reyes, tangled in muck on the banks. The newspaper photo makes him look like a skinned reptile left for dead on the rocks.

The stratified recreation areas inside Santiago parks are successfully pruning daytime desire. It's no longer so easy to slip in a squeeze under the public eye, and so city dwellers will continue to seek the lapping cover of darkness for reigniting human touch.

NEW YORK CHRONICLES
(STONEWALL INN)

And if they invite you to New York all-expenses-paid to attend the anniversary of Stonewall, twenty years after the police beat-em-up in 1969 starring gay chicks who took over a bar in the neighborhood known as the Village. And if they tell you the tale and you feel obligated to cross yourself three times at the place where it happened. A dingy bar, sanctuary of the homosexual cause, where the sodomites from out of town come to lay their floral offerings. Because there behind the windows hang tattered photos of the hippie veterans who resisted the law's assault for who knows how many days—the police who aggressively tried but failed to dislodge them. So why not shed a tear in the gay Grotto of Lourdes, practically a religious shrine for the thousands who respectfully remove their Calvin Klein visors and pray a few seconds while lining up for the dance club next door. Why not fake at least one Hail Mary if you're a visitor to these parts and they're staving off your hunger and paying for everything, these militant holier-than-thou gringas who commercialize their political history. Why not politely pretend to be overwhelmed by those faces in black and white—as if it were some old movie we just never happened to see. These photos of gay heroes who look like they're straight out of Woodstock, crowned in the window with roses and colored ribbons, same as the whole block, same as the whole Village neighborhood, decorated like one big cake in the full regalia of fairy fashion. Because when you come up from the subway at Christopher Street, you're hit in the face with two tons of muscles and bodybuilders in minishorts, waxed and with pierced ears—male couples in roller skates who whiz by holding hands as if they don't even see you. And why should they, you being so awfully ugly and having dragged your third-world malnourished loca body all the way here. Why would they give you the time of day, with that surprised Chilean face of yours before this Olympus of beefy, virile homosexuals who look at you in disgust, as if to say: We're doing you a favor, little miss native, bringing you to the cathedral of gay pride. And you go stumbling around these scenes from the Great World, looking at the shops packed with sadomasochistic fetishes: nails, sharpened hooks, clamps and screws for ruining your complexion and torturing your tuchus. Ay, what pain! What a fright to see that group of Leathers on the corner with their motorcycles, mustaches, boots, and a fascist brutality that reminds you of the macho gangs in Chile whom you're careful to give the slip, crossing the street and hurrying past while pretending to look the other way. But here in the Village, in the square across from the Stonewall Inn, this masculine virility abounds, causing you to panic, making you shrink until you're only a little bug from the tropics that's landed in their neighborhood of blond sex, in this part of New York, the pink zone where stuff costs an arm and a leg, the commercial epicenter for gay tourists who visit the city. Especially now, during these global festivities, when the island of Manhattan is draped with flags sporting all the colors of the gay rainbow. Which really is just one color: white. Since maybe gay is white. It's enough to step into the Stonewall Inn, where it's always night, for you to figure out that the majority of the crowd is white, blond, and lean, like saloons in old cowboy flicks. And if by some chance there's a Black man or some Latina loca, it's just because no one wants to be called antidemocratic.

Which is why I didn't stay very long in that historic bar—a quick look around and you'll see you don't belong here, that you have nothing to do with the postcard gold of its muscled, classical aesthetic. New York City has other nooks and crannies where you won't feel as strange—other, more contaminated places, where the Latina soul salsas its territorial song.

CHILE: SEA MEN AND CUECA
(OR, "GET DRESSED, JUANA ROSA")

Winter's freezer having only just begun to thaw, leaving behind a deathly August that caused the elderly to bundle up in terror as it passed, the spring reaches us, bringing with it another September curdled with cocky Chilean-ness, snaking through the air along with bursts of pollen and pink clouds of plums.

A chilenidad dripping in the syrup of honeybees, labeled as "sweet homeland" or national marmalade. Like the cotton candy that children eat in O'Higgins Park, which sticks to their hands and faces along with the dust kicked up by the military's goose step in the parade. Or the sweat of the fat lady who seasons the ground beef for empanadas with the sopped wattle of her forearms while she wipes boogers from the baby who lets out a wail to the beat of the cueca's whoo-wees and whoopsie-dos. Or more like the merengue and salsa that have replaced our boring national dance, which is no longer a dance at all but just a mathematical choreography for TV. Gaucho aerobics where twirls and macho harassment spin a woman into submission.

The cueca is a dance that reenacts the Spanish conquest of the Amaricón cowboy in his little flamenco getup. A two-piece suit brimming with buttons, and matching boots with fringes and a butterfly heel. The estate's ranch hand who poshes up like a proper flirt with a jacket cut at his waist to show off his little ass. The rodeo cowboy who chases the china all the way to the henhouse. And the china is the servant girl who soaked her braids in Temuco's night sky. The china is the nana, as the rich now call the girl they keep on hand. They don't tell her *arréglate, Juana Rosa, que te llegó invitación.* They tell her she's a service girl, because on the Eighteenth of September she'll have to wait on their many guests and so won't be able to put on lipstick and meet up with her sweetheart in the park for a stroll beneath the trees. Instead she'll eat a rancid empanada alone in her minuscule bedroom, fingering her white jacket and the garish flowers on her polyester skirt and her high-heeled shoes that made her chubby legs a little longer. The swarthy candor of her eighteen years, knowing that on this and all future Eighteenths she'll rot away in the same servitude.

And so the national holidays spur forward with their ruckus of red white and blue piñatas. And so vendors gamble their loose change on a business that sometimes tanks in a storm, every plastic flag, paperboard cowboy hat, and golden pinwheel dragged into its current, the colors fading like imagined winnings in the September betting rings.

Even so, between the mud and the speakers that crackle and hiss with gurgling water, the more it rains, the more people drink. A healthy man really has no excuse, already depressed that he's a worker with a miserable paycheck, that he can't share even September Eighteenth with his main squeeze, Juana Rosa, who had to stay behind to clean up her bosses' vomit. La Juana Rosa with her shy heart, like a southern songbird, who must be feeling awfully lonely in her cage while the rest of Chile uncorks themselves partying. And between the onion belches and soused vinegary barrels of homemade chicha con naranja, we keep gulping until we die. Or at least until we forget chilenidad and its opportunistic grasping. Forget the president's laugh and the military generals' five-star grimace that merge in tricolor spittle over our shared nips of chicha.

Drink to forget other, nightmarish Septembers, other cuecas danced with bare cold paws over scattered glass from the window smashed in by a soldier's knife. We're still drinking to anesthetize the memory, until the bodies pulsing on the dance floor to *muévelo, muévelo* blur with the glass fogged with alcohol. And after seeing so many tits and swaying hips in the sawdust of the ring, the body wants a shake. It doesn't matter how the dance goes, simply step into the dizzying nausea of so many people moving together. Join the party beneath the shoddy tent that's already brimming with peepers, just like your bladder ready to explode if you don't take a piss. And in the early morning frost, somewhere between *excuse me* and *mind if I . . . ?*, behind the refreshment stall platforms, the bubbly stream lets loose, forming a chorus with the row of other weenies squeezed to bursting from so much celebrating. And someone at his side, pretty young from the looks of him, asks: Want me to get you off? And he's so lonely and bitter this Eighteenth that he doesn't think twice but just gives the boy a wink of assent. And the teen hangs on to his willie like a suckling calf, provoking a wave of tenderness that makes him stroke the boy's gelled bangs, mussing his hair in an ejaculating outburst and murmuring: Take it, chilito, eat it, it's all yours.

And while the cumbia's humming and the accordion's grinding out *mira como va, negrito*, and hurried joints are smoked in a tumble of embers that for a second illuminates the boys' faces, he falls, rolling down the ellipse of the park in a topsy-turvy of baton twirlers, meat skewers, cocks, and posters of Mother Teresa, Verónica Castro, the Pope, the Colo-Colo soccer team, and all the saints who have been canonized by roadside merchant hawking. There he lies, flung out on the grass, his open fly revealing his willie lolling like a drunk snake. Out of money because the sipping fairy nicked his entire paycheck as payment for services rendered.

The national holidays are like this, an effervescent inertia that unites our yearning to belong to wherever we are. To be at least a hair on the tail of a taxidermied Patagonian deer. Or the pointy tip of the star, anything that whiffs of Chile in order to feel at ease and munch on scraps of the barbecue that wafts only so many times a year from working-class backyards. For a few days, they stucco the buildings' sallow complexions with color, draping the passageways and their dusty revelry with garlands.

The plebes get their tiny allowance of happiness, which flutters in the flags they sew out of uneven fabric scraps. As if the sheer amount of proletariat red in this misshapen geometry might maroon that unreachable blue. As if that same roiling purple could then migrate into the white, chafing it into a violent rose. Playfully turning the flag's pure colors into a flower stained by the rust on the walls.

It would seem like this ignored class of people should be laughing at this identity that's been forced on them, transmitted via government trichomoniasis. As if the state, through these patriotic carnivals, were desperately trying to shore up the voice of a people whose culture was lost somewhere in all the Aiwa cassette players that sing on the street corners with Andalusian hoarseness, Mexican wails, and rock 'n' roll lyricism.

A supposedly shit-faced identity that hangs its hat on these flimsy symbols instead, which at this point in the century are imported from Japan, like patriotic birthday decorations that glow just briefly, on certain days of the year. And once the euphoria ends, the brightness of that same September sun fades away, returning the city's inhabitants to their commutes, as they make their way back to work, a little bit sadder, their shoes worn out from dancing.

WHERE THE MUSIC AND THE LIGHTS NEVER WENT OUT

Like any other Saturday that pricks the city streets, hoping the night explodes in a sweet boozy nothing of music and dancing. Just in case some runaway heart turns up, reflected in the gay nightclub's mirrors. It's still early for a night out in the port city, but the madhouse is already burning at Club Divine, everyone churning their hips to the dangerous beats of Grace Jones, whose "La vie en rose," with her flaming African tongue, takes us for a ride down the French Riviera inside a sports car upholstered in ermine. Inside that pansy fantasy of jet-setting in Marbella, or Cannes, dancing to the same music, splashed by the same lights, and rummaging for loose change for another pisco and Coke so they don't get too glum while looking out at the dirty port and its mildewed canisters. Another cola for the loca drowning in Old Spice, please. Another spin of Grace Jones on the dance floor, showing off the secondhand Calvin Kleins, which look new if you iron them right. Especially in a darkness shattered by spotlights. Pray that the music and lights never go out, that the cops don't show up asking for ID, that nothing goes wrong on this magical night that feels like New Year's Eve. Pray that everyone keeps dancing and that the disco's pisco fairies keep running their hands over each other in the corner. That's why no one notices the smell of smoke rising from the stairwell, which makes an asthmatic loca cough, who says she has a loca's poor lungs. Someone shouts, *Turn up the fla-ame!* Turn up your whole oven, honey, but don't let anyone turn out the lights; not even the glow from the firebomb that a fascist just hurled at the door. This lustrous yellow that climbs the steps like wildfire, which upon reaching the travestis' wilted plumage ignites the crazy glue in a shower of purple sparks, and everyone breaks into applause as if it were all part of the show. But whatever, the music and the lights don't turn off and Grace Jones keeps singing, which is why no one takes it seriously. How could you know the front staircase has collapsed in a thunder of ash with the music so loud and everyone sweating to begin with? What difference does a little heat make if the locas are hot to trot and on hearing *fire! fire!* there's always one who will say: *Where? Here in my heart*. But seconds later the joke goes up in smoke. As if the lights and music were playing along with the Dantesque scene that burns behind closed doors. Too hot to keep dancing, too terrified to rescue the Levi's jacket in coat check. Crushed together like kernels on a cob, the locas shouting, pushing, trampling a gasping girl who was choosing to die from fright. Looking for the back door, the key nowhere to be found. *Try the bathrooms!* says someone who once saw this in a movie. Braving their way across the bright coals of locas on the dance floor, still twisting to Grace and the music that keeps thumping. Stepping over beams and red-hot mirrors refracting Nero's Roman discotheque, the overhead speakers stoking the bonfire. Not looking back at the gay couples already mummified in Pompeii's ashes. Seeking refuge in the false chill of the bathroom's plastic tiles. Like choosing lust's own turf in these last moments, remembering frenetic scenes and quick sucks, reliving in the middle of an emergency the moist air and wet sex of Movieland bathrooms. Quick, run all the taps instead, in every sink, but the paltry drip that comes out is boiling hot, and the smoke fills the throat of an asthmatic loca who doesn't want to die. An asthmatic loca who claws at the tiles that burst into tongues of flame. An asthmatic loca who smashes the mirrors, putting out the fire's reflection, at least. An asthmatic loca who, finding an exit with a last mouthful of oxygen, doesn't know if her life or her lungs suffocated her more, who knows she's going to hell and so wants to live no matter what, burning her hands, clambering up the smoky scaffolding until she finds a window on the third floor, so tall, so high up. And with such a big audience below, waiting perversely to see if she jumps into the void, over this crowd of onlookers who will watch fires without caring what happens. Deciding to take the leap because just maybe she'll float down on the golden air that's now burning her lungs. Daring to do it now, since she's already burning and the sea's so far away and a vertigo of waves is applauding her. Barely a step, the bonfire pushing her from behind as it ignites her hair into a torch. One step, a single step on a glass runway, and the spectacle of a loca in flames, flying high above the Valparaíso docks, will be remembered as a glittering jewel on the city's prostituted neckline. Because, even then, even though the police claim that electricity short-circuiting is what caused the fire—the music and the lights never went out.

Discotheque Divine, Valparaíso,
September 4, 1993.

EVEN POPPIES HAVE THORNS

For Miguel Ángel

On weekends, the city streets flood the libido, getting young bodies high on the usual desires, which, depending on how early or late it is, might be cash or just relief from a vicious boredom that sometimes leads them to swap a virgin forest's curly leaves for the damp tunnel of urban-anal passion.

Those fraught couplings shroud the sidewalks where locas hooker in search of an impossible heart, vampiring the night away under bridges, in back alleys, and in parks, where the darkness is a black sheet that smothers their sighs. The loca is the night's accomplice in the gray light of abandoned lots, where it's easy enough to purge that horniness, that fever let loose on a Saturday night when bored boys from the outskirts descend on the city, looking for a mouth to suck them and even throw a few pesos their way.

The loca knows where these adventures end, sensing that what comes after will be something awful, especially on a night like this one, so charged it might explode. Something in the air warns her, but also turns her on, the whiff of degradation mingling with the music. That urge of who the hell knows. Ay, the gnaw of being a bitch in heat, an anal hysteria that never lets her sit down. Ay, what a clamor. Ay, this hemorrhoid tingle that alcohol sets on fire, like a stray hot coal pushing her, clandestine and alleywayed, out onto the street.

The homosexual seems to possess a certain courage in this infinite capacity for risk, tucked in the shadows, tossing her glove like a party streamer at the first macho who winks back.

As if testing the usual roles, infecting their borders. Disrupting the image of a gay couple and their hybridized wedding bouquets; seducing one of those hard boys instead who on the first drink says never, on the second probably, and on the third, if there's a fag, it'll be blown somewhere outside in the downy scrub.

That's why the loca's night smells like sex, an unknown something makes her roam through the streets looking at forbidden fruit. Her fairy eyes slide down, linger only a second, piercing between the legs, right where the jeans are an oasis distressed by the zipper's groping. A quick glance, batting her eyelashes in fluttering complicity with the boy, who looks down, frowning, thinking he left his fly open. But no, and yet that sharp pupil pricks him right there. Then he figures out this piece of him is worth its weight in gold to the loca who keeps walking and discreetly turns her head to watch him. Three steps more, she pauses in front of a shop window, waiting for the playboy to catch up and ask her sidelong: What are you up to? Just walking. Let's walk, then. What's your name? It doesn't matter, everyone's a Claudio or a Jaime when following a loca who promises them a good time. The playboy adjusts his bulge and makes nice, hoping they're headed to a huge apartment with tons of whisky, music, and a nice bit of cash at the end. But he's stuck with only a cheap cigarette, and after going in circles in search of a dark corner, they finally wash up at an abandoned lot littered with trash and dead dogs, where the loca frees her tarantula across his erect denim tent. There, wrapped in her fiery fingers, the little tough guy relaxes into the genital rocking of this queer suckling calf who murmurs: Put it in me for a minute, just the tip. You want it? And without waiting for an answer, he pulls down his pants and plugs it in himself, thrusting, sweating into that burning hinge, and she whimpers: Ow, it hurts, not so hard, it's really big, slow down. You like it, I'll split you in two, eat it all, I'm going to come, I'm coming—don't move—oh, I came. And just like that the boy spills his hot milk on the rear tourniquet until the last drop sperms his groan.

Only then does he look at her coldly, as if from one moment to the next whatever was forging his disillusionment has cooled and condensed into a dirty mist that now spreads over the lot, a nuptial bedsheet for the loca who panting asks for "a little bit more." Her pants still around her shins, she offers her velvet magnolia smeared in the rennet that blossoms her each night. Her slice of heaven cracked open, split in two and horrific, oh won't a hungry ass come eat the petals, playing he-loves-me-he-loves-me-not. Come and water her homofagous flower dribbling lace and sodden seed-crowns in the clench, her late-night gynoecium incubating young saplings. Her carnivorous pucker sprouting them in fecal ardor. Her prickly poppy straining forward, an open slit still unsatisfied. Emptied by lack, a black hole gnaws at her insides, a gnaw of knowing the wrinkled thing that retracts into its French-letter flap. Like a wasp who abandons the corolla, having sucked the honey out of each membrane, and turns back toward the dump's familiar stench. The feasting over, her empty chalice rehollows post-partum. Her withered sphincter shines with absence, a pupil that blinks unseeing between two cheeks. Even if it was a waste: a one-eyed conch, a blinded oyster, a clammy mother-of-pearl who lost her jewel at some point during the party. And all that's left is a faint trace of it, like an anchovy radiating an iridescent memory across a pile of trash. Its gleam stands out against the dim streetlamp that casts a shadow across the boy's folded wee-wee, a sad pendulum that sheds a final tear, yellowing the boy's boxers right as he flees, catching the bus while he's still splattered with blood. Asking himself why did he do it, why did he become so disgusted with himself, that sour bile in the back-and-forth over the loca's wristwatch: It was my mother's, the loca said, pleading. The loca who squealed like a hog when she saw the blade, that harmless pocketknife he carried around just for show. And he'd never cut a soul in his life, but that loca screamed so much, it was unreal, and he had to skewer her again and again in her belly, in her eye, in her side, so she'd finally fall down and shut up. But the stubborn fag wouldn't fall down or shut up no matter what he did. She kept screaming, as if each thrust gave her more life, more energy to leap and prance with his puppet who was dancing death. Because she sucked the knife like a dick, begging for more, one more time, Daddy, that last one nearly killed me. As if the dagger were an electrified prod and its discharges just tightened her flesh, stretching her, exposing virgin territory for another stabbing. New parts of her body exposed in the poses and theatrical gasps of the loca's agony. Trying to cover her face, ignoring her underarm torn open at the tendons. Slashed in the kidney, the loca pulls through, still on her feet, channeling Monroe in the flash of the cuts, doubling over like Marilyn for the Polaroid shutter of the pocketknife that opens the chamois of her flank, modeling gash after gash of disembowelment fashion. A major star in a fresh display of entrails, receiving the silver comb like a trophy. Practically "mahvelous!" she catches the metal as if it were just an accident, a light scratch, a rip in the Christian Dior gown styling her purple. The trannie mannequin flaunting a classic look on the red carpet puddling beneath her, burlesque in the muah of kisses she trades for a flash, ironic as she offers her ravished lips to the fist that will shut them for good. The boy's hard again, the finger inside his pants a blunt point pincushioned to the bright red carnations that bloom on his chest. The rag doll of a loca who resists effetely, lifting the macho's dispassion to new heights. Holding in her vomit of copihues, she flirts with him; leering wanton into the bullring, she defies him. The night's barren land is now the smooth silk of battle, the bullfighter's kerchief that turns scarlet in a single flamenco twist. The red bubbling out of the maricón's wounds transforms the boy from the slums into a real Andalusian gypsy. He is the topaz matador who cuts her in two, lilies her in her bubbling liver, the slashed angel of Seville. Our Lady of Sorrows in all her hemorrhaged finery, menstruating in the bullring, mortally wounded as she bellows up crimson and weevils, crying uncle, begging for a truce, a break so she can find the drunk stab of the dance's rhythm again. But the little boy, newly erect, tears petal after love-handled petal from her flesh. He lynches the fag to infinity, cuckolded by his own churning confusion. Up the ass, up every failure, every kick from the pig cops, every spit that she returns with a bloody kiss, saying through clenched teeth: Don't you wanna lil bit more?

The next morning the headlines write themselves. The incident doesn't cause a stir, because moral judgment agrees with what happened. It endorses the front-page cruelty that says she got what she deserved: HE WHO SEEKS SHALL FIND; KILLED BY HIS OWN RULES; STABBED FROM BEHIND; and so many other clichés that the homophobic tabloids use to twist the knife even deeper.

Public opinion will focus morbidly on the fact that locas tend to hang around these areas. Forgotten plots of land that the city then breaks up, building developments over the ashes of the crime. But the violence against homosexuals in these dismal theaters goes way past a brawl, a robbery, or an act of revenge. They are butcheries where society's resentment demands the weakest, most vulnerable hides—the gypsy hearts of locas who seek a drop of pleasure in the thorns of a forbidden rose.

WILD DESIRE

Fording gender's binaries, giving the old sepia family photograph the slip, and above all picking the pockets of scrutinizing discourse—exploiting its intervals and silences—halfway and half-assed, recycling oral detritus like excreted alchemy: wiping, with a gossip rag, the pink smudge of a sphincteral kiss. I abide the unpleasant aroma to appear before you with my difference. I say in my minoritarian way that some groove or marrow etches itself into this constrained micropolitics. Cramping from camp, dis-ass-emblable in stripteased faggofication, reassemblable in straight obliques, politicizing toward sissy self-knowledge.

I expel these excess materials from a doughy imaginary, dolling up political desire in oppression. I become a beetle that weaves a blackened honey, I become a woman like every other minority. I yoke myself to its outraged womb, make alliances with the Indo-Latina mother, and "learn the language of patriarchy in order to curse it."

Parodying patriarchy's rectitude, obliquing myself once again inside the haunts and hair salons of travesti sisterhood. Plucking from our feathers any inky quills that tried in vain to explain us. So that at least we wouldn't get depressed feeling utopia's breezes. Because we never participated in those liberationista causes, doubly far from May '68, submerged in a multiplicity of segregations. Because the sexual revolution that today is stuck back inside the status quo was a premature ejaculation in the third world's back alleys, and AIDS paranoia threw the homosexual's progress toward emancipation out the window. That wild desire to assert yourself in a political movement that didn't exist—it got stuck between the gauze of precaution and an economy of gestures dedicated to the sick.

Which has little or nothing to do with the hospital that shipwrecked on our fraying coast. A gay movement we didn't participate in, and yet we catch its deadly hangover. One of the developed world's causes, which we eye from a distance, too ill-iterate to articulate a stance. Too feminine, too much flipping our hair and flirting with power. Too busy keeping our penises out of work to worry about anything else.

Cloistered inside our filthy ghettos, sewing fabric scraps for the underground clubs or seducing a townie on the scratched velvet of movie theater seats in a two-for-one matinee. While in Valparaíso they beat the travestis on the dock and herded them onto ships, General Ibáñez and his cruise ship of a horror movie playing forever in our memory.

But no one believed it really happened, and, in the end, those bodies frosted over with bruises were just the ordinary refuse of an aristocratic homosexuality that flipped through imported fashion magazines looking for pictures of the international gay parade. Imagining themselves in California or emptying their piggy banks to join the euphoria. So far from this illegal reality of crimes that go unpunished, slashed travesti girls dripping red ink across the newspaper, a pale punished face there for all to see, like one more stab into the silvery stateless betweens of her ribs.

Corpses and more corpses weave our story into a cross-stitch. A string of scars embroiders the rough satin insignia into a smoky halo that blurs the letters together. Class separates the locas, homos, and travestis from the comfortable gays who scramble up the social ladder.

Doubly marginalized for our loca desire, as if it wasn't all enough already, the kicks from the system, the insults that claw at us daily, the utter indifference from not just the politicians but also those reclaiming homosexual power, which we see only as a speck in the distance.

Unable to wrap our poor Indigenous heads around the gay century, terrified of making a scene. Maybe we didn't want to understand and escaped just in time. Too many social clubs and associations full of serious macho types. Maybe we were always crazy; crazy like the women they stigmatize.

Maybe we never let that imported discourse precolonize us. Too linear for our madwoman geography. Too much blond militarism and golden musculature that then succumbed to the horrifying crucible of AIDS.

So, how do we take charge today of this project? How can we form our own cause, transforming ourselves into exotic satellites of the groups created by white majorities who find our feathers endearing; who organize their massive congresses in English, so our Indoamerican tongue can't have an opinion about how they organize their politics. We're treated like younger siblings, right down to our Indigenous stammer. We nod without understanding, the flashy whirlwind of European capitals making us self-conscious. They pay for the flights and the rooms, show us their civilized world, annex us in the name of their dominant pedagogy, and, when we leave, scrub our muddy footprints off their wall-to-wall carpets.

How are we supposed to see ourselves in the gay aesthetic, blue and tortured, all those nipples stuck through with safety pins. How to align ourselves with these forniphallicated masculine symbols in chains and leather, with all those sadomasochist fetishes. How can we deny maternal mestizaje with these representations of force that are now considered masculine, forming misogynistic parallels with power.

Gay fastens to power. It does not confront, does not transgress. It offers the category "homosexual" as a regression to gender. Gay coins its emancipation in the shadows of "victorious capitalism." Gay can hardly breathe in its necktie noose, but nods and squeezes its weak backside into the coquettish space that the system provides. A hypocritical change of spheres just to make another orbit around power.

Maybe Latin America—marked by reconquerings and transfers of power, with culture cross-dressing the wounds (covering, graft by graft, the brown skin of its own moon)—blooms in a warrior faggofication that wears tribal cosmetics as its marginalizing mask. A bodily militancy that speaks from the very edges of its voice its own fragmented discourse, whose most vulnerable sector, lacking rhetoric or political ground, must be homosexual travestismo, the underclass that finds its way into the darkest folds of Latin American capitals.

Maybe the only thing that can be said, the only writerly pretension that can come from a body politically unincorporated into our continent, is a babble of signs and common scars. Maybe a lost glass slipper molders in the vastness of this ruined field, somewhere among the stars and sickles buried in its Indoamerican hide. Maybe this political desire can zigzag, skimming along the top of these clearings. Maybe this is when the running stitch of modernity becomes the seam or side that breaks off, the weave of its theories tearing to reveal a South American validity in the homosexual condition, won back from serfdom.

COUP

FOR FIVE MINUTES YOU BLOSSOM

(VÍCTOR JARA)

The sky on the morning of September 12 was somehow dark, a slaughtered gloom over a Santiago still waking up from a bad dream, a sleepless nightmare of gunfire barking all night long. Armored trucks heading for the capital drove down the Panamericana firing rounds, scattering groups of neighbors who were out on street corners trading news about the coup. The spring air thickened into clots of zinc over the housing project roofs, over the kids playing cops and robbers, shooting their little hands at the helicopters that circled in a sky flustered with doves. In stairwells and alleyways, a commotion of old women who back then weren't so old, more like young women, middle-aged, hanging laundry from their balconies, still fresh in the floral polyester of their housedresses. Tough women, who cooked and cleaned and didn't understand what was going on but looked worried, pointing in their gossipy way with their lips and eyes to the throng of neighbors in the distance, which wasn't distant at all, barely half a block along the slum that added color to the vacant land between the Panamericana Sur and Avenida Departamental. Right here, where today they're building a gas pump and a resort for government employees, there used to be a trash heap known as The Pit that in the mornings reeked of rotten dog, a deep quarry where they dug out sand and gravel, the dump where garbage trucks poured out the city's rotten insides. In this small mountain range of filth, the children from the housing projects would play ski on the trash slopes, using a metal tray to slide down the dangerous hillsides of steaming roof tar. We hunted along these scummy urban cliffs for small treasures: gold foil wrappers, toothless emerald combs, a page from *Ritmo* magazine stuck beneath the spine of a dead dog, a blue bottle of magnesia dripping with fresh poo, a shiny chunk of vinyl record, half-buried, reflecting the silent music of a trash heap swarming with flies, worms, and rats on that morning in September 1973.

Three cadavers could be seen from the building's top floor—on the fringes of rubbishland, still tangled in their final breaths, their bluish flesh still warm, the early morning mist sprinkling them with dew. What I saw, on that morning from my childhood, as I poked my head between people's legs, was three men splattered with iodine, my neighbors speculating that maybe, like the television had been reporting, they were delinquents after all, executed during the state of siege. They noticed that the oldest man lying there had been wearing a toupee, but that it slid off when he was bashed in the head, revealing his cracked-open skull like a handful of rubies coagulating in the sun.

Something about it didn't make sense to me—"delinquents" didn't seem to fit those forty-five- to sixty-year-old bodies, those gentlemen wearing plain sad clothes ripped by bayonets. Maybe uncles, fathers, grandfathers, mechanics, electricians, bakers, gardeners, union workers, arrested at the factory and finished off right there, at the rubbish heap in front of my house, so far from the families who'd waited up for them with their hearts in their throats, holding a hundred years' worth of vigils in a single endless night, never to see them again.

Twenty-five years have passed since that morning, but the same shiver still runs down my spine every time I remember those twisted mouths, full of flies; those shoeless feet; those socks darned and ripped again, where cold, bloated toes poked through. The image has come back to me again and again, across time, *como un perro que no me deja ni se calla*. It's slowly become familiar, the visual sensation of seeing their freezing coffin plush with trash. I could almost say that, from my childhood's fetid scrublands, ripening under a moon of black pearl, their contorted hands greet me with fists in the air, the fruit of a bitter harvest.

PISAGUA ON POINTE

And only today, when the country has leapt into the future, lugging a knapsack of cadavers that drip blood onto the path of truth and reconciliation. When the days of terror have all but evaporated into the past's menstruated halo. Nights of doors banged open, mornings with olive-green trucks outside the house, waiting for passengers on their way to banishment. Heading south, to an island left off the map. Heading north, to an abandoned saltpeter mine turned into a concentration camp. And right then, in that moment when the soldiers are forcing them to go, holding machine guns and shoving the new detainees who, hysterical, leaving behind their pasts, their homes, their families, have no idea what to throw into exile's suitcase. Grabbing a sweater, a scarf, and a coat in case it got cold. But, José, don't forget your pills. But, Carmen, your needles and insulin. Plus socks, undies, and sanitary napkins for the girl-woman arrested at school. In the rush, not knowing what the future would hold, where they were going, it was hard to predict what to pack for exile. Especially if given only a few minutes, troops pushing and shouting at them as they rounded up leftists beneath the dismal green canvas of armored trucks.

On the morning they came looking for Gastón the choreographer, his house was a jumble of clothes and bundles that his twirling dancer hands tied and untied. Photos, makeup, leotards, and ballet slippers were strewn across the floor, while he—a ballerina who'd worn his heart in his toe shoes for Allende—reached for a scarf, threw out a set of silk pajamas, selected a jacket, wondered about taking a polo shirt, packed some high-heeled boots, knocked a hairbrush to the ground, as two exasperated soldiers pointed their guns at him, fingers on the trigger. Do you know where they're going to take us? asked Gastón, arching a waxed brow. That's a military secret that can't be discussed. Hurry up, we're going to be late, barked the conscript. But I need to know if it's north or south, if it's going to be cold or warm, to see what clothes I should bring. I think you're going north, said the soldier gruffly. But what part of the north? Mountains or beach? They said Pisagua. That's waves, beach, sand, and sun, thought Gastón, grabbing his bathing suit and a towel on his way out.

And so, on those long afternoons in the concentration camp, facing the sea in Pisagua, while his fellow inmates argued in long political meetings to which he was not invited, while the other prisoners carved handicrafts or penned secret resistance poems if the guards weren't watching, when the yellow sun glared off the turquoise blue of the waves, the figure of Gastón sunbathing in a Speedo on his orange towel, barbed wire framing him in the distance, was practically an advertisement for tanning lotion amid that landscape of isolation and death. The slumbering dancer's image must have been a strange contradiction, banished twice over on his square meter of sand, exile, wire fences, and watchtowers where the guards laughed at the summer holiday he was taking in that jail beneath the stars. But really it was Gastón who was laughing at depression and just how serious it was, being in that prison. It was the only way to escape, even if that meant bronzing himself flamboyantly on the same ground that would later become the mass graves in the north.

You can't be such a fag here, Gastón. We're in a concentration camp, buddy, not on the beach in Rio, his bunkmates reproached him, an edge to their voice. And what was I supposed to do, if you guys spend the whole day in meetings and more meetings and there was such a pretty sun hanging over the sea?

Minorities sometimes come up with other ways to act in contempt, using what seems like superficiality as a weapon. Gastón, tanning on his beach towel, knew how to break free from that yard of torment, as if a loca's irreverence could transform a beach towel into a rug for flying, a magic carpet that would hover over the iron bars, float out past the soldiers' guns, and raise him above that camp of horrors.

Maybe some of the prisoners who got out of there alive still remember the morning when Gastón received his letter of transit, granting him permission to depart immediately for exile in some European country. Gastón, grinning from ear to ear, carefully put away his bathing suit, folded his towel, and breathed deeply, gulping down air as if he wanted, with a single sigh, to erase the morbid atmosphere of that place. Then he wished everyone goodbye and, walking on the tips of his toes, crossed over the spikes at the entrance. And, still glowing tropically, he disappeared from the road in a cloud of dust, never looking back.

IF YOU DON'T RETURN

Who could have known that I'd pine for the rest of my life, like in the cheesiest kind of music, those kitschy ballads for sappy women and lonely aunts, the pulp songs that sometimes howl out from radio programs. And it was weird that you, of all people—a tough kid from La Jota at that public academy where we were both enrolled in high school during the Popular Unity years—actually liked those schmaltzy melodies. Even more confusing was that, me being an obvious fruit basket case, you were the only one who would kick the ball into my corner at lunch, risking mockery. *Pues la ciudad sin ti . . . está solitaria*, you never stopped singing under your breath with a resigned laugh that, to make things easier for you, I never shared. I heard that song again recently, all these years later, and remembered how much I'd admired your revolutionary candor back then, loved your cheerful commitment that became fury when you heard that fascists were planning to destroy the Ramona Parra mural on the front of our school. We have to guard it all night, you said, but no one listened because we had a test the next day. Who cares about the test, you think I give a rat's ass, I'm staying here to watch over the people's mural. And I didn't care about the test either when I snuck out of the house at midnight and took off toward school, and I found you nestled there clutching a cudgel, standing guard under the mural's birds, raised fists, and hungry mouths. *Pues la ciudad sin ti . . .* you laughed, surprised to see me, scooting over so I could sit next to you. You couldn't believe it, and you looked at me and sang, *Todas las calles llenas de gente están, y por el aire suena una música*. I came to keep you company, comrade, I said, stammering out of shyness. Your company would be welcome, comrade, you replied, passing me what was left of a joint from your juicy lips. I don't smoke, I said chastely. So I didn't smoke, didn't breathe, didn't sniff, didn't drink, only loved with all the furious passion of my sixteen years. The fascists might come. You're not scared? I said no, trembling. It's the cold, I said, it's really cold tonight. You didn't believe me, but hooked your arm around my shoulders with a warm squeeze. *De noche salgo con alguien a bailar, nos abrazamos, llenos de felicidad . . . mas la ciudad sin ti . . .* It was weird that you'd sing this song and not something by Quilapayún or Víctor Jara, which your party comrades all strummed. You sang it slow and low, as if afraid that someone might hear. It's just . . . it was as if you were singing only to me. *Pues la ciudad sin ti . . .* you hummed each verse against our tense night of kiddie vigilance. By your side, I almost didn't feel the cold, and, talking slowly like that, about so many things, our naive sufferings, I became more and more relaxed, dozing off on your shoulder. But the sound of someone approaching cut my breath short in terror. Don't move, you whispered in my ear, raising your stick. It might be the fascists. And we stayed like that together, our hearts beating *dum dum*, waiting. But it wasn't the fascists, because the footsteps disappeared, echoing out from the empty street. And then we were alone in the quiet. *Y en el aire se escucha una música*, you began to sing again in my ear, and the hours went by like that, and the next day we both flunked, and then came final exams and our schooldays sprawled into marches protesting Vietnam and meetings in support of President Allende. And then all of a sudden the music cut out, the coup came, and its brutality made me forget that song.

I never knew what happened to you. Winters passed, their storms washing up cadavers in the Mapocho, all of them shot through the head. Winters passed with a kerosene stove and the TV tuned to Don Francisco, his burlesque little theme song the background music for the dictatorship's wooing of the country. Everything was like that, all imported fanfare, with busty chorus girls sitting on the generals' laps. The only music that echoed in the streets after curfew was the military's showbiz sirens.

I never knew what happened to you: maybe you were in hiding, or snatched away, tortured, riddled with bullets, or disappeared inside our national pain's musical score, which is silent and without justice. Something tells me it was like that. Santiago is a street corner, Santiago is not the big wide world: here sooner or later everyone finds out, everything comes to light. That's why today, after hearing that song, I mouth it silently just for you and walk splashing through puddles in the park. This winter is coming on hard, the fall afternoon sinks into a sky reflected off pools of water. Cars jammed together honk their horns at the traffic lights. The students come and go with their enormous backpacks, ready for the cold or some big march. The city dwellers shove each other at the bus stop, waiting for the Transantiago in a mass, in chaos, in a tumultuous commotion that saturates the streets. *Mas la ciudad sin ti . . . mi corazón sin ti . . .*

MERCI, BEAU COUP

And this all took place in a simple country, strung from the cordillera and with a wide view of the sea. A country drawn on the map like a loose thread, like a sluggish salt snake that woke up one morning to find a machine gun pointed at its head, as nasally broadcasts repeated: "All citizens must return home by curfew and avoid the terrorist hordes."

It happened in the first months after the Eleventh, during those blowout parties celebrating the coup's thwack, while the neighbors were still busy rescuing people and hiding people and saving people and fleeing along with them. Some military genius decided to organize a charity drive to help the government. The idea, surely copied from some Nazi pamphlet or *Gone with the Wind*, called upon the Chilean people to donate their jewels—replenishing government funds and rebuilding our national patrimony, which Unshaved United had all but drained, so said the blonde dames over their teas and canasta games, organizing fairs and raffles to help dear Augusto come out ahead in his heroic efforts. Showing the whole world that the coup was nothing but an electrified spank on a naughty boy's ass. The rest was pure libel and slander from foreign communists, who frankly were jealous of Augusto and the other generals for knowing how to put their pants on and finish off an orgy of hobos in a single smackeroo. Well, then, if you wanted the coup, go ahead and declare your support by contributing a little ring, a necklace, whatever you can. Go donate a brooch or one of your grandmother's jewels, said Mimí Barrenechea, the admiral's wife, gussied up as the campaign's most energetic promoter of gifts of silver and gold, which she graciously accepted at a gala thrown by ladies in pastels who ran around like clucking hens receiving the offerings.

The military government presented them with a tin pickaxe as a token of thanks for their historic contributions. The country is in ruins after spending so much on troops and bullets to take back our freedom, added Mimí, goading filthy rich women into trading their wedding bands for a copper ring that would soon stain their fingers green as a moldy emblem of their sacrifice.

The gala drew reporters from every news outlet, though all they really needed was *El Mercurio* covering it and Televisión Nacional broadcasting the rich and famous as they lined up to hand over a diamond necklace passed down in the family like a holy chalice, national inheritances that Mimí Barrenechea scooped up tearfully, saying to her aristocrat friends, This is what being a patriot means, duckie, and screeching joyfully to these same varicose vixens who'd been by her side banging pots in front of the regiments, the same ones who'd helped out at the Military Academy cocktail parties, the Union Club, and even in la Mimí's very own home, adding up their millionaire alms to help the army. That's it . . . right over here, Consuelo . . . I'm coming, Pía Ignacia . . . la Señora Barrenechea sang as she filled baskets stamped with the national crest, and at the sound of her upbeat, priggish step in fell the trinkets of platinum, gold, emeralds, and rubies. With her dreaded sense of humor, she parodied Eva Perón as she yanked jewels from the necks of her more reluctant girlfriends. Ay, Poochie, weren't you so happy about the coup? Didn't you clap and drink champagne on the Eleventh? Then hand over that little ring which looks like a wart growing on your arthritic finger. Give me that pearl necklace, dear, yes, the one you're tucking under your blouse, Dust Bunny, turn it over to the cause.

Then, Señora "Bunny" Larraín, miffed, touching her bare neck, which had just lost this exquisite necklace she had loved so much, replied: And you, dear, what are you contributing? Sensing that everyone's eyes were now fixed on her, Mimí looked taken aback. Ay, Bunny, I've been running around so much for this campaign, would you believe I completely forgot? Then set an example with this expensive sapphire brooch, said Bunny, grasping Mimí's collar. Remember that charity begins at home. And in horror Mimí watched her enormous blue sapphire, which her granny had gifted her because it matched her eyes, flash as it fell into the charity basket, taking with it her nationalist volunteer spirit. She felt terribly depressed as the basket of gemstones moved on, and for the first time she wondered what they would possibly do with so many jewels. Whose name was on the bank account? When was the auction, where would it be, so she could rescue her sapphire? But even her admiral husband couldn't tell her, and he scowled, asking if she doubted the army's honor. And so Mimí kept her doubts to herself, though she never did see any accounts or report about how much their encrusted efforts had raised.

Years later, when her husband brought her to the United States for work and they were invited to a reception at the Chilean embassy for Pinochet's newly appointed Lady Ambassador to the United Nations, la Mimí, wearing gloves and a gown, arrived on her admiral's arm to a ballroom full of uniforms sparkling with medals, gold brocade, and decorations that tinkled like Christmas tree ornaments. But all she saw in the glare of golden stripes and shiny buttons was a blue flash at the nape of the ambassador's neck. Mimí stood frozen at the top of the marble staircase, her husband tugging at her arm and clenching his teeth as he said under his breath: What's wrong with you, stupid, come on, everyone's staring at us. My-sa, my-saph, my-sapphi, stammered Mimí, her eyes glued on the smiling ambassador who was approaching to welcome them. Say something, you idiot. What's wrong with you, her husband whispered, pinching her so that she'd greet this woman who looked heavenly, dressed in cornflower-blue silk with that diadem trembling at her scruff. My-sa, my-saph, my-sapphi, repeated Mimí, about to faint. What's that? asked the ambassador, not understanding the babbling Mimí, who was hypnotized by the jewel's sparkle. It's your brooch, my wife likes it a lot, replied the admiral, bailing her out. Ah yes, gorgeous, isn't it? The commander-in-chief has such good taste; he gave it to me as a gift. He presented it to me with such a heavy heart, you know, explaining that it was a family heirloom, said the diplomat, touched, before moving on to greet the other guests.

La Mimí Barrenechea couldn't get over the shock, and that night she drank everything she could lay her hands on, even the dregs in the glasses the waiters were clearing away. Embarrassed, her husband had to drag her from the table, because for la Mimí getting drunk was the only way to dull the pain. She needed fix after fix so she wouldn't crack, so she could bite her tongue and not say a word, not a single peep while, her vision blurry from the alcohol, she gazed at her lost jewel, its brilliant surface refracting the coup in all its splendor.

BLACK ORCHIDS

(OR, THE DINA'S CULTURAL CENTER)

The parties, overflowing with guests and dripping with whisky, were thrown at what was the swankiest house in Lo Curro, back in the midseventies. Where amid the dictatorship's fraught airs music floated through the open windows, Proust and Faulkner were read with devotion, and a set of highbrow gays fluttered around la Callejas, the hostess. Mariana Callejas, a literary diva who'd sunk her anti-Marxist roots into the Patria y Libertad quagmire. A woman of restrained gestures and steely gaze who, wearing black, charmed everyone at the literary salons with her mettle of an army sergeant and her adorable pout. A woman whose good breeding and short stories made her the young promise of Chilean literature. Even the leftist magazine *La Bicicleta* published her, and she was lauded and praised by the bohemian elites, the cultural class who showed up to her parties back then, so self-assured, who didn't believe those stories of dead bodies or people who disappeared. No, they gave the whole thing the slip by reciting Eliot, debating avant-garde aesthetics, and wiggling their skeptic asses to ABBA's beat. Entirely intoxicated by Mariana's macabre orchids.

Many familiar names filed through that little house in Lo Curro at each afternoon literary soirée, where these artists and writers were served tea and scones, or whisky, caviar, and Camembert whenever a really famous writer visited, who'd wax poetic about the house nestled in greenery and the landscape of the Andean foothills and those birds breaking the neighborhood's necrophiliac silence. The peace and tranquility of a crypt, just what every writer needs, complete with a garden of jasmines and honeysuckles "to cover up my husband Michael's laboratory, he's a chemist and always up late working on a gas to exterminate rats," Mariana would say with a pencil in her mouth. Then everyone would raise their old-fashioneds to toast Michael Townley's exterminating elixirs—his swastika labors that gave off a real stench, withering any roses that crept too close to the window.

It's possible that these guests didn't really know quite where they were, though almost everyone knew those unmarked cars, the vulture's silent flap. Those taxis that picked up passengers only after curfew. The whole country knew and kept its mouth shut, everyone had heard something, something was said, some piece of gossip or cocktail tidbit about a censured painter. Everyone saw but chose not to look, not to know, not to listen to those horrors that leaked in through the foreign press. Bloodstained hooks and electrical sockets upholstering dark rooms, twisted bodies in mass graves. It was too horrible to believe. Those things don't happen in such an advanced society, in a country of writers and poets—sheer sensationalist aesthetics, "sheer Marxist propaganda to discredit the government," said Mariana, turning up the music to drown out the strangulated cries coming from the garden.

After Letelier was killed in Washington and the investigation into his death exposed Lo Curro's secrets, the artistic highfliers couldn't get away fast enough from that house they'd visited so many times. Many received notices from lawyers in the United States, inviting them to testify, but they all said no, scared off by threatening phone calls and the obituaries slipped under their doors.

Though Mariana became a cultural pariah, unleashing terror whenever she showed up at literary rituals, she still retained, for years after the fact, a few gay pearls on her string of admirers. She continued to exercise a grim power over ardent fans of the short story, who once even invited her to the Society of Writers, in their not-so-secret house on Calle Simpson, full of political posters, ponchos, berets, and those protest songs that Mariana, seated in a corner, listened to indifferently.

Everyone there knew what she was capable of, this woman who feigned an interest in long poems about torture. Everyone was on edge, wondering who invited her, avoiding eye contact so they wouldn't have to shake her hand and receive the light electrified charge of her touch.

Surely anyone who took part in those cultural soirées of post-coup kitsch will remember how the voltage would spasm and how annoying it was, interrupting the dancing, making the lights flicker and the music skip. Surely no one knew about the other dance going on below, where a metal prod would twist, drawing tortured backsides into voltaic arcs. Possibly they couldn't tell whether a scream wasn't just part of the dissonant disco music, all the rage back then. So they were just stupid, then, comfortably stupefied by cultural cachet, by whisky the DINA paid for, and by the house, too, an innocent little house with two stories, where literature and torture mingled together in the same drop of ink and iodine, in a bitter, raucous memory, smothering all vowels of pain.

WHERE WERE YOU?

And if they've told you everything was fabulous in the eighties, kid, that we'd all go down to the Omnium to sip cocktails with our lacquered bangs and those idiotic clothes they advertised on TV . . . If they've told you this decade was a fashion blockbuster, that the babes were all dead ringers for Bolocco and wore shoulder pads like Farrah Fawcett, that the boys danced to Jackson and Depeche Mode in Club So-and-So in the fancy part of town and that they'd strut around Apumanque Mall in their acid-wash jeans, that they watched some gringo movie over and over and how much we all loved *Charlie's Angels*, that we were all little blond imbeciles dancing to the beat of marching boots. Don't believe it, kid. Luckily, there was another Chile, eighties ista and Allendista, where being an artisan was all good, where using wool from Peru was dissident and decent, where wearing a dab of patchouli oil and dying your hair purple was a secret code. Because we had to counteract that fifteen-years-of-fame gang that filled the TV slots. So bienvenido woolen hippies and artisan fairs where Silvio would play on cassettes, slow and low. Bienvenido Hindu clothing and long hair, real long, dreamed down to the waist in my eighties utopia. And, hidden from the police, we'd smoke Los Andes joints and feel that we were protesting all that Chileanish shit others loved so much. There was rock, too, way before Los Prisioneros, there was always rock growing under the stones, surviving the dictatorship. Groups like Tumulto, or Arena Movediza with its furious Zeppelin metal ringing out from the Klimax Disco on the south side of the Alameda. This was before Matucana's counterculture and underground scene. Just a few beatnik poets reading their verses in dark canteens. There we lived in our tiny truncated territory with its tearful seventies emotions. And what else . . . everyone else was somewhere north of Plaza Italia, at right-wing parties after curfew. Nothing ever happened to them, they didn't walk around holding their ass in both hands, plastering up posters of Neruda. They didn't even bother to step outside their bowling alleys because they were grossed out by all the woolen university students who armed themselves with Molotovs, their eyes red from boxed wine. That's how it was, old homeboy who now wants to insist on his boring and empty eunuch memories.

The eighties began from below, with whispering flutes and sad guitars. There wasn't anything to celebrate on that stage of crimes and tortures. There was no reason to party beneath the glaring stage lights of *Sábados gigantes*, that pinochetista television show. It was a gagged, fearful, and sour country that watched Maluenda cheer on the armed forces on daytime TV. The old cardboard hypocrite Maluenda who broadcasted the regimented cueca. Who now appears in the movie *Tony Manero*, almost like the director was paying homage to his early remember-me-chilena. Yuck, the fatherland vomited copihue flowers back then. *¿Dónde estabas tú?* sang Los Jaivas, and today I'll ask you the same question. Where were you? Even if you make a thousand films about the dictatorship, we won't forget that song. Tell me, where were you? There's an eighties you didn't live, and it's too late for cinematographic explanations. Memory is a snail that closes up inside its unforgivable shell. It happened just like that, us here and you there, as if the tyranny didn't exist. Always joshing about, blowing bubbles in your Tom Collins in the Casa Milà Pub, the Hollywood disco and all that jubilant shit. We were bitter and we were afraid. We also danced, we flew, and sometimes we were happy, but our happiness stung with rage. We were mobilized by wrath. Disco pulsed from the radios, with Canto Nuevo in the canteens. The eighties came like a comet, burning a bloody free-for-all, the first protest, the student movement, destrangulating the fear, fuck. There was also rock, there was always rock and marijuana, green and pressing. Not to be confused with the preppy little misters who made themselves into rebels on TV, singing the regime's pop and rock ballads, rotten hams not worth remembering here.

"The era is giving birth," a mop-top centrist strummed—while we listened to Violeta breathing on our strung-out cassettes. These were the beginnings of a decade rife with political twists and turns, a decade we'd never forget, unveiling its rages in that armored dawn.

RONALD WOOD

For that rumpled blossom of a boy

Maybe there's a way to rescue Ronald Wood from being yet another young person whom the eighties riddled with bullets. Maybe we could meet his honeyed gaze somewhere in the many empty sockets of dead students who'd dreamed a future too bright for this unjust democracy to bear. When I think of Ronald, a memory of him as a grown child hits me in the chest, and I look up at the clouds, squinting to make him out in those blustery celestial bedsheets. When I mention him, I struggle to picture his smile rotting in the ground. When I dream about him, his absence salts the vast blue of the sky, and I struggle to believe that his playful whirligig gestures won't be there to greet me in the morning.

Because wouldn't it be nice to see Ronald again, in Maipú, where I worked as an art teacher during the iodine rodeo known as the seventies. And Ronald couldn't have cared less about art, goofing off the whole hour, spilling paints, staining the clean sheets of paper in his fury, distracting his tidier classmates. While I was flipping through slides, trying to teach them about cave paintings. While I was showing them Egyptian art, handing around laminated images of pyramids and pharaohs' tombs. And Ronald, indefatigably hyperkinetic, bored with my educational yakety-yak, would sprawl in defeat, his adolescent legs grown suddenly long. Because he was the tallest, the bothersome dunce too big for elementary school benches. The class clown who made teaching a torment, drawing all over his face, laughing at my discussion points—until we reached the Romans and their empire's military art. Then, for the first time, I saw him sit up, staring with disgust at the sculptures and busts of emperors and generals, the friezes depicting tyrant armies. For the first time he sat still, listening, and I used that flicker of interest to slip in some politics—risky in those years, when it was a sin to speak about current events in the classroom. And Ronald paying close attention, participating, helping me in this shared subversion through the unlikely means of our visual art unit. Later, after class ended, when everyone had trooped off to recess, I glanced up from my attendance book: Ronald was the only one who remained in his seat, silent. And what are you still doing here? Didn't you hear the bell? He looked at me with his enormous chestnut eyes and, without saying a word, stretched out his arm to offer me half his schoolboy apple, like a heart split in two, sealing our secret pact.

From that day on, his beautifully rumpled self hung on to every word of my anti-military lectures. Hey, prof, he'd say under his breath, we've gotta do something to end the dictatorship. We're doing something, Rony, don't get ahead of yourself. Meanwhile, you need to study and set a good example, not go around breaking the detention hall windows and sticking your tongue out at the principal. Understood? And I'd leave him there, in the middle of a yard scarecrowed with children, lost in thought, scratching a head of hair so blond that it gleamed like a lemony flame in those distant crystalline mornings at the end of the seventies.

But my strategy of radicalizing with classical art didn't last long. At some point something got out, someone heard, and, without being told why, I was forced to quit teaching in that district. I never saw Ronald Wood again, had no idea what happened to him in the strained years after that. I never found out whether he, too, had been expelled from the school.

Only on May 20, 1986, did the news reach me that he'd been killed in a student protest on Loreto Bridge. I figured out only that day, from the newspaper, that Ronald had been studying to be an auditor at the Professional Institute of Santiago, that he was barely nineteen years old on the afternoon when a sneaky little military bullet blew out the kindling flame of his passionate life. The article said that he spent three days in agony after the dictatorship's lead had shattered his gorgeous brow.

But for years I swear I'd catch his laughter in the gaggle of students stirring up the parks and plazas, the river, the warm spring afternoons. Some part of me is still not convinced he's really gone, and I keep picturing him blossoming in the yesterday of his mottled pubescence. Perhaps I'll never fully dispel the guilt that clouds my memories of his big hazel eyes and those distant public school days, when he handed me the other half of his red heart.

NIGHT AT THE CIRCUS

According to my dear amiga Andrés Pavez, who just passed away, this happened to a loca who was always cruising the streets for a bit of dirty dancing, who one September evening ignored the terrifying curfew that our octogenarian fatherland had set. Ah, those dictatorship Septembers, full of holidays and commemorations and barricades and glorious protests under repression's strained skies. But our loca never let a little political unrest get the better of her. Especially on that particular day when, gathering her savings, she went out to buy a pair of those fancy brand-name sneakers she'd been dreaming of, which cost as much as an eye from your face. But it was a luxury she could give herself, walking real posh from Central Station on down, at the cusp of national paralysis, the hour when everything in the country froze. The perfect hour for catching a wayward macho for a rubdown in some empty lot. And she walked springy in her shiny Adidas as people ran past, catching the last bus home by the seat of their pants. She strolled fresh in her winged Adidas as people hurried along, neurotically checking the time. Santiago turned tough once the streets emptied out and the only sound after dark was the screech of police sirens making the city's heart race. In those days certain ladybirds, hungry for ass-fuck express, liked to comb this Santiago set on edge by curfew in search of fresh semen. And that was part of the challenge, the dangerous loitering, snagging something right before time was up. Well, the loca in her spanking Adidas drifted down the Alameda, on the west side, unable to find anything, not a single soul she could squint at in the night's hairy silence. But a ways off, near General Velásquez, she could see strings of shining lights announcing that the big circus had come to town, as they always do during the holidays, pitching their tents on the empty land by that central street corner. And so the loca steered herself that way, pulled by the glowing signs, and arriving, found only more endless solitude, with just five minutes to go before curfew. Got a cigarette? She was startled by the gruff voice of the circus hand, who guarded the tents. Oof, finally something, sighed the loca in relief. And then by the light of the match she caught a lusty glint in the macho man's eyes, and without any chitchat he lifted the door on the canvas tent where he slept on a field cot. His foldable bed was the only thing there, and why bother with more? thought the loca, untying her gorgeous Adidas, which she placed delicately on the floor. Then she surrendered to the orangutan clamor of this man, who ate her alive, skewering her again and again with his circus tent pole. Such frenzied sexual contortions wore out the mighty man, who, having gotten it out of his system, immediately began to snore. That's it, the loca said to herself, silently getting off the cot to look for her spanking Adidas in the dark. And she looked and she looked, groping under the bed, but couldn't find even a trace of her footwear. Then she realized the tent was a bit short and didn't reach the ground—and that if someone had seen the shoes from outside, they'd only have had to stretch out a hand while she was busy with sodomite combustion.

It was certainly a tragedy to have lost her flawless Adidas, but it was even worse to have to leave after curfew, in the wee hours of the morning, with bare paws. Snooping around under the bed, she thought, There's got to be something around here, something I could wear, even just old flip-flops, and then she felt something like her sneakers, but so big . . . and pulling them out, she found herself with a pair of enormous clown shoes. Well, what can you do, she said, strapping the pointy boats on her queenly little paws. Being very careful, she went outside, shuffling along until she reached the circus entrance, where she hid behind a sign for a while after hearing a patrol car's motor. When the silence returned, she dashed across the Alameda, conking like a stampede of circus animals. She stopped behind a tree on the other side of the street, waiting until the echoes of her sprint had faded away. And so the loca went, clowning into the night, from tree to tree, running and stamping, hiding and trembling, as she crossed the besieged city with her heart in her hands and her dirty little bum leaking onto the dictatorship's gloomy streets.

FLASH ART POLITICS: THREE TALES

EL COORDINADOR CULTURAL

If I don't tell the story here, it might get lost, as memory twists and closes like an oyster around *remember when*. Because the eighties had barely begun, and those days were so grim and blighted there was almost no light, and only a few of us voiced our outrage in public, through demonstrations that tried to wake the Chilean people from their sleepwalking, their consciences struck dumb by marching boots. Here and there, in disguise or on the down-low, actors, painters, poets, and political groups would meet up after curfew to plan acts of sedition against the regime. And that's how El Coordinador Cultural was born—a ragtag committee of activists and artists who staged interventions on politically symbolic days. I think it must have been for September 11, as by sunrise the streets were already policed, just like every year, ready for any hint of protest. The organizers had met beforehand, in an unknown location to make sure the details weren't leaked, which meant the exact time and place where we would intervene were kept secret until the last possible moment, the instructions passing only mouth to mouth to avoid using the phone or writing anything down.

What I'm describing sounds like a movie set in Nazi Germany, but it really was that risky: the cops had shown up at a previous action, arresting people and beating them, and someone had died. The spot on this particular Eleventh was the plaza across from the Municipal Theater—a pretty dangerous choice, being right in the middle of downtown. But the organizers had placed a team of medics and some lawyers about a block away in case anything went wrong. It was never clear how many of us would show up, but many people risked it that day. As we pretended to wait for the bus or passed by each other quickly without saying hello, we realized we were almost a hundred total, each acting as if the others were strangers. Everything would start when the cannon fired at noon, and it needed to be simultaneous and extremely fast. The moment the cannon blasted from the hill, near the theater on Avenida San Antonio, an actress appeared in the crowd, holding a blue balloon (this was the signal). She was carrying an armful of packages, and they tumbled to the ground as she crossed the street, causing a commotion. While other pedestrians helped her pick them up, a vehicle drove into the intersection and a bunch of familiar faces jumped out, forming a chain to cut off traffic. Then the flash action really began: everything had to last no more than three minutes. This was how long it took for the cops to arrive from Paseo Ahumada, a couple blocks away. The painters ran with watches in hand, pasting signs about the dictatorship over the opera's posters. The poets hurried to the statue of Mekis, the sleazy mayor, on the corner of Bombero Salas, placing money bags in his hands along with a sign that said WATCH ME RUN OFF WITH THE CASH. My job was to dye the water in the plaza's fountain across the street. I'd hidden the bags of red earth in my floral backpack and pulled them out in a huge cloud of dust that I threw into the basin, but the color clumped at the bottom without the desired bloodying effect. A street sweeper stood beside me, watching the whole scene gobsmacked. Give me that broom, I said, grabbing the handle and quickly stirring the red coloring. Just in time to get the hell out of there—a group of dancers were still trying and failing to lift a sign in the air with bunches of balloons, but as soon as we heard a whistle we took our exit.

Oof, what a time, what emergencies we lived through, risking ourselves like that to protest. It's strange, but there aren't many who remember anymore. The details have disappeared along with the protagonists, back when no one thought to stage something so public. There weren't too many of us, after all, maybe fewer than a hundred, who converged that day at noon, with our ass in both hands and a lustrous sigh electrifying our lips.

A TREE FULL OF LEGS

When one casts out the line of memory, episodes begin cropping up, episodes that for a long time no one wanted to remember, since forgetting was safer. Maybe El Coordinador Cultural wasn't meant to last longer than a flash of lightning. And no one ever documented these actions of taking over the city with political art, with art that made theater a form of rebellion. We didn't have video cameras or any of the technology that is easy to find these days. I don't remember the exact dates, but they were important times for the Left. As always, the precise location was kept secret, and our instructions were to bring long pantyhose stuffed with paper, plus an empty package inside a bag. So that's what we showed up with that morning, on the corner of Irarrázaval and Bustamante Park. We strolled around, circled back, saw a few of our companions, whom we could spot from their homespun woolen sweaters, pretending to be sweethearts. We barely looked at each other, averting our eyes as we passed. This time around, again at noon, a car appeared, tossing pamphlets and a Molotov and a tire into the middle of the street, creating a line of flames as a barricade. The traffic came to a halt. The action began. It was an open space, which meant we had to be more careful. Someone could shoot at us from the park while we stood there, in the middle of the street, hurriedly pulling out the stockings crammed with paper to look like legs. Flesh-colored stockings that resembled severed limbs, a huge pile of legs pulled from some authoritarian mass grave. The idea was to hang them from a giant tree in the park, as if they were human fruit swinging from the branches. A resistance poem painted on a huge banner crowned the scene, though I don't remember what it said. All of us clambering up the trunk, all of us desperate, tying knots in the pantyhose as the tree bloomed calves and muscles and feet that winter morning. And if I'm being honest it wasn't nearly as artistic or surrealist as I make it sound, because in our rush the legs were hung badly or fell onto the grass. We didn't have art's rigorous, ceremonial pause for pulling off the performance. The police could appear at any moment; Pinochet's secret service could drive up and shoot us dead in the street. Besides, we still needed time to vanish into thin air, which is why we then dropped our heap of packages and boxes in the street to throw them off. It was all a matter of minutes (*la vida es eterna*): some graffiti, some shouting, some honking, some pamphleting, and book it up Irarrázaval like you farted. And after walking quickly for quite a few blocks, hop onto a bus that, as luck would have it, makes a U-turn and circles us right back there. We watched from our seats as the whole police apparatus arrived—surely some neighborhood toad had tipped them off. They prodded the mysterious packages with a pole, thinking they might contain a bomb. And the traffic remained at a standstill, with all of us on the bus with our stomachs in knots, praying the police wouldn't board and search the passengers. But they did, of course, squinting at each of us with suspicion. Let's see that backpack. Señora, open your purse. And you, what's in that bag? But they didn't find anything. So the bus started up again, and the tree of legs was behind us, looking lyrical and tragic from far away. Yes, the tree was behind us, blossoming with legs that the police were already ripping down. That's it, really—just flashes of street art for the resistance that were gone in the blink of an eye. There aren't any photos of these actions that helped keep our spirits up, softened a bit of our rage. We replayed the day as we headed home. How young we were in our efforts for the sickly homeland, delighted to be the perpetrators of a minor offense. We didn't even tilt the brim of the tyrant's hat, let alone make the news. Everything kept going—the country didn't alter its fenced-in course. Meanwhile, El Coordinador Cultural was planning its next action. This time it would be a call for a nationwide strike. And we'd need to do something that everyone would see.

EVERYONE ON STRIKE!

The fact of the matter is, El Coordinador Cultural was at the forefront of the art activism that emerged from that decade. Not all of us were artists, and the actions weren't all that highbrow, more often they were a lot of shouting and dashed-off broadsides after a particularly gruesome event. The dictatorship was as nasty and murderous as ever—and only a nationwide strike would be able to undermine it. So this would be the call to action, the igniting moment.

We had to keep switching up where we met, and there weren't many options. Studio 666, the Mapocho Cultural Center, the Society of Writers—but these places were too smoked out, too closely watched already to risk a police raid. Which is how Studio El Sol—a peña, a homespun cultural center—became the place where we prepared our big action to kick off a nationwide strike.

We would make an enormous sign announcing the strike and float it down the Mapocho River, a raft of resistance for the city. It was a more limited, guerrilla operation for being so dangerous—the sign would be huge, and had to be built out of wood and plastic. Plus, it had to float on inflated tire tubes. I was the one whose job it was to buy those tubes at the flea market. And it wasn't easy to walk down the street carrying a heap of tires during the dictatorship. But scared to death, I did it.

There were twenty of us, dressed as a construction crew with overalls and yellow helmets. Our story would be that we were workers hauling this rolled-up, sixty-foot sign on our shoulders. We'd throw it in the river at Puente Los Carros, in La Vega. It could have been September again, I'm not sure, but we'd spent the whole week painting and putting together this giant sign that said simply: EVERYONE ON STRIKE! We'd have to attach the floats, as fast as we could, while we were on the bridge. The whole business was suicide, no question. The time was set for noon, like all the previous actions.

That day we met at eight in the morning in Studio El Sol to get organized and receive our instructions. The group was made up entirely of men, so as not to look suspicious, and of course there was another gay besides me—someone from MIR, who's now dead. I won't use his name because he never came out as a homosexual, though he was aware that everyone knew. He was a writer who focused on oral history and eyewitness accounts. There was nothing at all affected about him—he was just very serious, and he never smiled. Now I remember him and understand his mute message: those weren't times to be fagging about in a protest. He was intimidating, with a deep voice and penetrating gaze. One time at Bar El Castillo in Plaza Italia, a poet had reproached him for being a homosexual, and, looking her straight in the eye, he asked: And what exactly is your problem with it, my friend? And she had to swallow her words. Then he went back to drinking his beer like nothing had happened.

The morning was tense, and we had lookouts watching the bridge in case there were cops. It was always possible that the plan would somehow get leaked. At eleven o'clock we all counted off and were ready to carry our enormous seafaring pamphlet. Which is not to say we felt at peace—a frozen calm began to drip down our spines when one of the lookouts showed up, warning us that the whole place was swarming with cops. Some women had strung a banner from the railing of the same bridge, and the cops had blocked the route off. It's impossible now, he told us, smoking a cigarette, troubled. We all looked at one another in disappointment, except the gay guerrilla, who stepped to the front, scolding us for being cowards. All the more reason to stick to the plan. I'm prepared to take the risk, he announced. The other men lowered their heads, muttering: I have kids, I have a family. Then the gay guerrilla became indignant and spat on the floor. We all have a family—it's because of them that I insist we carry this out. He looked so determined, standing in front of this group of machos in costume who refused to cooperate. Which of you will take the risk? he asked, looking at each one of us. But he was met with silence. And then the reckless loca in me jumped out, and, stepping to the front, I said: I'll risk it. Who else? Who will join us? And we stood there alone, just me and the gay guerrilla in the breach as the machos retreated, a little ashamed. We were two stubborn faggots who didn't have any backing, and we couldn't carry out this dangerous mission alone. It's already noon. Who will join us? the gay guerrilla asked again. At that moment, someone started banging on the door, breaking the silence. We all scrambled, trying in vain to find a way to escape. The sign, the sign, shit, grab the sign. The patio, the patio, drag it out to the patio and hide it on the roof, we whispered in desperation, pulling the huge roll out of the room and raising it onto the roof, trying to make as little noise as possible. Someone looked in through the window and opened the door. And our souls flew back to our bodies when we realized that it was just a chubby friend of ours who'd run all the way back from the bridge. The street's full of cops, he panted, collapsing into a chair. And that ended everything. We undressed slowly, removing our helmets and overalls, and I took the chance to get an eyeful of my guerrilla compatriot's hairy legs.

This was the failed, final action of El Coordinador Cultural and its brief history during our volatile dictatorship. I've shared it here so that my reckless memories and their tattered petals don't get scattered to the neoliberal winds.

AIDS

DIAMONDS ARE FOREVER
(FRIVOLOUS, CADAVEROUS, WAYWARD)

Everyone in the homosexual ghetto knows who's positive. The rumors spread quickly—a purse opened in a rush, strewing papers and medicine across the floor. There's always a snoop who helps pick everything up as she asks: And this medical certificate? And so many bottles and pills? And these syringes, honey? Don't tell me you're an addict.

Wherever the campy bacchanal briefly roosts—preventative programs, marches for recognition, cultural events, fashion shows, hair salons, and nightclubs—there's always the insinuator, the gossip, the knockout puncher who shrieks when she sees the suddenly pale face of a friend come through the door. That sarcoma looks fabulous on you, girl! And so the sick are taken for healthy and the syndrome's stigma becomes another one of the club's features, a chummy familiarity that makes the drama feel like no big deal. Or it's that addressing the epidemic in this way might be the only cure for depression and loneliness, which are what end up destroying the infected first.

At one of these faggified parties, everyone overheated and half-delirious, it's easy to find a positive loca who agrees to answer some questions on the subject, avoiding what you usually get in TV interviews: the Christian pretense, the masculine tone of voice the sick adopt in front of the cameras so they don't end up doubly ostracized. Here playing instead with the disease's celebrity aura, subverting the AIDS testimonial, the humiliating interrogation where the homosexual carrier is always standing on the dock of the accused.

Q: Why carrier?
A: It has something to do with letters, with what arrives at your door.

Q: How so?
A: Well, my door is gated, but not like a prison or a fence. It's a garden gate covered in flowers and little birds.

Q: Baroque?
A: I don't know what that is, but maybe so, the iron grating's covered in cardinals.

Q: And where does it lead?
A: To the garden of love.

Q: The gate opens?
A: It's always wide open.

Q: And what's inside the garden?
A: A chair, made out of the same iron, matching the gate covered in—

Q: . . . flowers and little birds.
A: And also hearts.

Q: Broken?
A: Yes, a little, a crack here, a fracture there, but no arrows. That whole thing about a cupid angelito is a hetero story. Instead of arrows, syringes.

Q: Oof, how awful!
A: Why awful? These days the pricking turns me on.

Q: Fine, but we were talking about love, the gate to the garden of love. Aren't you avoiding the subject?
A: Always, they should never know what you're thinking.

Q: And what are you thinking?

A: I don't think, I'm just a talking doll, like those Barbies that say *I love you*.

Q: You speak English?
A: AIDS speaks English.

Q: How so?
A: You say, *Dahling, I must die*, and you don't feel it, you don't really feel what you're saying, so it doesn't hurt, you're just repeating gringo commercials. But for them it hurts.

Q: And for you?
A: Almost not at all, there are many things worth living for. AIDS itself is a reason to live. I have AIDS and that is a reason to love life. Healthy people don't know why they should love life, and every minute escapes them, like leaky pipes.

Q: Is it a privilege?
A: Absolutely, it makes me special, seductively special. Besides, I have everything guaranteed.

Q: How's that?
A: Look, as a carrier I get a doctor, a psychologist, and a dentist, free. I study for free. Anyone who hears the whole sad story immediately feels sorry for me and says yes to whatever I ask for.

Q: Except for love.
A: Well, it's true, people would like you to die, so that they feel safer, more alive. But us carriers, we're beyond love. We know more of life, though we get it at a discount. Right this minute, I'm happier for knowing there won't be another.

Q: There's never another for anyone.
A: But it's different for me. You're going to watch it snow someday, if you go to Farellones or somewhere else rich people go. But I never will, because I might already be gone. And the snow always melts before I arrive. I have the same dream over

and over again: I reach out to catch a snowflake, but my hand only touches water. You see? Something's always leaving.

Q: Like a race against time?
A: My soul evaporates before it gets there.

Q: Like in that song?
A: Exactly, but without the music. Desires, wishes—we're trying to hold onto them.

Q: And what about growing old?
A: Ah, there's another guarantee for you. I'll never be old, just like the stars. They'll remember me as young forever.

Q: And if they discover a cure?
A: I'll die anyway, because who knows how long until it arrives in Latin America, or what the price will be. Can you imagine how much it's going to cost? The rich will be saved first, like always.

Q: Like AZT.
A: Yes, but as I see it, AZT is like silicone: it stretches you out, plumps you up, makes you bigger, maybe adds a few months to your life. Some travestis inject it themselves.

Q: AZT?
A: No, silicone. I once met a travesti at a bar in Talca who told me she had everything but gas for the plane. And I thought she meant AZT. No, honey, she said, for my tits. And how do you do it? In a clinic, I imagine. Are you kidding, I don't have money for that. I buy two bottles of pisco, drink one, and when I'm good and sloshed I take a razor and cut myself right here. Look, under the nipple. There aren't too many veins there and you don't bleed as much. And? Well, the silicone, it's like gelatin, right? Like those sea jellies you find on the beach. So you stick it inside the slit and sew it up afterward with a needle and thread. And the second bottle of pisco? You throw it on the wound and drink the rest. You're stitched to death,

but afterward the silicone falls forward and covers the scar, you can't even notice. See?

Q: This was in Talca. Is there a lot of AIDS there?
A: As much as anywhere else. There the travestis call it *the shadow.*

Q: Come again?
A: The shadow struck, that's what they say. It's a pretty expression, mind you. Like eyeshadow. Notice how all of us who have AIDS, we have looks that kill?

Q: Forever . . .
A: Notice how something slips away when you stop looking at me? Something breaks. Look at me.

Q: I am looking at you.
A: No, you're not looking at me, you're looking at my death. Death took a vacation in my eyes.

Q: Why so much poetry? Does it soften the drama? Make it easier to bear?
A: Look, I'm not talking about being poetic. More like being possessed.

Q: And do you write?
A: Sometimes, on these hot, sticky days most of all, when it's just about to rain. I'd like it to be raining when . . . when my hour arrives. Flowers always last longer in water.

NIGHT OF FURS

(OR, POPULAR UNITY'S LAST SUPPER)

Santiago swayed with earthquakes and political tidal waves that were breaking apart Allende's young coalition, Popular Unity. The air carried whiffs of gunpowder and the endless clanging of pots and pans that the rich ladies beat in time with their bracelets and jewels. Blonde dames shouting for a coup d'etat, a military takeover to put a stop to the Bolshevik scandal. The workers watched them and grabbed their crotches, offering sex, before bursting into laughter, all with rows of freshly cleaned teeth, all free as the breeze they happily breathed while waiting in line outside the UNCTAD building for lunch. A few locas wove their way among the workers, pretending to have lost their vouchers, searching in their crocheted bags, pulling out handkerchiefs and makeup until finding the slip with a little cry of triumph, their sultry glances and insistent caresses sliding between the men's sweaty bodies. All those proletariat muscles in a row, waiting for the lunch counter at the People's Cafeteria that distant December of 1972. Everyone was cheerful, talking about the latest episode of *Música libre*, the handsome Mauricio and his olive-pit pucker, his Romeo haircut. And of course his tight bell-bottom jeans that clung to his hips, squeezing their nosegay of hopes. Everyone loved him, and everyone was his secret lover. "I saw him. He said it right to me. I'm meeting him again next week." They egged each other on, making up stories about the kept prince of television, reassuring each other that he was one of us, that he, too, bit his pillow at night. Someone swore they'd bring him to the New Year's Eve party, to the all-you-can-eat bash promised by la Palma, that cracked loca who sold chickens at La Vega and who, wanting to feel herself a queen, had invited half of Santiago to her end-of-the-year party. And she said she was going to kill twenty turkeys so that the girls could stuff themselves and not leave wagging their tongues. Because she was happy with Allende and Popular Unity—Even the poor, she said, were going to eat turkey that New Year's Eve. And so word spread that her party would be unforgettable.

Everyone was invited: the broke locas, the Recoleta locas, the Blue Ballet locas, the locas from Carlina's, the streetwalking locas who cruised along Huérfanos every night, la Chumilou and her travesti gang, even the Coppelia queens and la Pilola Alessandri. They all met up on the UNCTAD patio to dream up the looks they'd unveil that evening. "The flowy shirt, the Saint-Tropez belt, the striped pants—no, even better, the wide ones pleated like a maxi skirt, with clogs and a mink stole on top," breathed Chumilou. "You must mean rabbit, dear, because I don't think you have any mink." "And you, honey. What color is yours?" "They're not mine," said Pilola Alessandri, "but my mother has two." "I'd have to see them." "Which, black or white?" "Both," Chumilou sniffed. "The white to say goodbye to '72, which has been such a ball for us poor faggots. And black to welcome '73, which seems to be coming on heavy, with all this racket of pots and pans."

And la Pilola Alessandri, who had offered the coats, was now stuck bringing them, and that night she showed up to the UNCTAD in a taxi, and after the hugs and kisses she pulled out the immense pelts taken from her mother's closet, saying they were real, her father had bought them at the House of Dior in Paris, and if anything happened to the coats she'd kill them. But the locas didn't hear her, wrapping themselves in the furs, modeling and striking poses while they walked to catch the bus to Recoleta, complaining that none of them had eaten a thing, least of all Pilola, who in her rush to take the furs had missed the family's splendid lobster and caviar dinner, so she was dying of hunger, her stomach in knots, desperate to get to la Palma's and taste that juicy spit-roasted turkey.

As the queens passed a police station, they picked up their pace, not wanting trouble, but the pig cops shouted for them to stop. So Chumilou turned around and, letting the mink stole slip down her shoulder, pulled out her fan and told them she was dressed for the night's festivities. On the bus afterward she couldn't stop playing stewardess, dragging the fur across the floor, singing a cabaret tune, transforming the ride into a show of laughs and saucy quips that distracted everyone from the oppressive summer heat. But when they arrived at the party, not a scrap of turkey was left, just a punch bowl with sangria and some half-eaten canapés strewn across the table. La Palma kept apologizing, running here and there because the queens had come, the famous ones, the crème de la crème who would suck their molars as they stepped off their planes. Those stiff-necked blondes who'd pretend they didn't know her on Huérfanos Street, the same glam locas who hated Allende and his party of popular undies, who shed strings of pearly tears because those scumbags had expropriated their mothers' estates. La Astaburuaga, la Zañartu, and la Pilola Alessandri—such freeloaders, such carpetbaggers, such visions of elegance in their mink coats. Because they came all the way to Recoleta on a bus, wearing mink like Taylor or Dietrich. No doubt about it. The whole neighborhood decamped to see them, those girls as sophisticated as movie stars, as models in *Paula* magazine. And the old townie ladies couldn't believe it, stood speechless watching them enter la Palma's house, this fairy affair she'd been planning for months. And to see them show up in furs, in such heat, looking around the house in disgust, saying sidelong, *such gorgeous dinnerware, honey*, meaning the plaster candelabras on the table, that sad table covered with plastic and littered with chicken bones and picked-over platters. Palma not knowing where to begin, trying to explain, saying again that there'd been so much food: twenty turkeys, champagne by the crate, salads, and every flavor of ice cream. But these cracked locas were so hungry, they left nothing, everything has been eaten. As if war were coming.

Cumbia and faggy cueca played all night long, splashing the first hours of 1973. As the party wore on, with the extra bottles of pisco and jugs of wine they'd sent the queens out to purchase, class nuances blurred in the clinking of glasses, in the hugs and warmth that unfolded in the backyard decked out with streamers and balloons. Ghetto alliances, shared seductions, cheeky hugs and ass squeezes from the neighborhood workers who stopped by to say hello to the pompadour queens, friends with the hostess. Gossip and shade that exploded into laughter and teasing over the absent feast. In the middle of a song, Pilola shouted, "Your turkeys flew off, honey!" and again Palma tried to explain, gathering the feathers and cleaned-out carcasses, showing them the cemetery of bones heaped on the table. At first the hostess blushed, red with shame each time the cumbia stopped and the queens shouted, "Catch that turkey!" But eventually, everyone was so plastered that the embarrassment turned into a game. All the locas began collecting the bones and arranging them in a giant pyramid on the table, like a mass grave lit by candles. No one knew where one of these witches had gotten a little Chilean flag that she planted on that morbid sculpture's summit. Well, that bothered Pilola Alessandri, who huffed and said that it showed a lack of respect for all those in uniform who had done so much for the nation, that this country was a populist slum thanks to Popular Unity, which had them all dying of hunger, that these flea-scratching locas knew nothing about politics and had no respect even for the flag. And that she couldn't stand to be there one more minute, so if they would please hand over her mink coats because she was going home. "What coats, honey?" responded Chumilou, cooling herself with her fan. "Us poor broads don't know such fine things. And in this heat? You'd have to be very stupid to wear fur, darling." The posh locas realized then that they hadn't seen their fine pelts in ages. They called for their hostess, who, drunk, was still collecting bones to build her monument to hunger. They looked in every corner, turned down the beds, asked around the neighborhood, but no one recalled seeing white furs flying over Recoleta's tar paper roofs. La Pilola couldn't stand it anymore and threatened to call her uncle the admiral if her mother's coats didn't turn up. But all the locas looked at her like she was crazy, knowing she'd never risk her honorable family diagnosing their son's cough. Declaring solidarity with the loss, Astaburuaga, Zañartu, and a few sympathetic upstarts also left, outraged, swearing never to set foot in this busted house again. And as they waited in the street for a taxi to retrieve them from those shores, the music blared out again from la Palma's house, pelvises began gyrating again, and "Mambo No. 8" signaled that the drag show had begun. Suddenly, someone cut the music and all of them shouted in chorus: "The minks flew off on you, honey! Catch that mink!"

The first dawn of 1973 was a faded chiffon over the open mouths of the sleeping fairies who were strewn throughout the house as if they had fainted. Cigarette ash on every surface, the streamers trampled beneath the garden overhang. Frustrated little groans rising from disheveled beds. Half-drunk glasses rocked by the rough tide of a quickie against the wall, smothered giggles remembering the minks' flight. And that shaft of smoky light coming in through the windows, wafting through the wide-open door. As if the house were a skeleton lit from above. As if the locas had conked out in this five-skull hotel. As if the candlelit pile of bones, still intact on the table, were an altar to what was still to come, a prediction, a year's horoscope that blinked black tears into the wax of candles about to snuff out, about to smother the last socialist spark out of the little paper flag that crowned the scene.

From that point on, the years tumbled like tree trunks in a landslide that buried the national fiesta. The coup hit, and the hailstorm of bullets made the locas scamper, never to dance again on the UNCTAD's flowering patios. They found other places, meeting up on avenues that the dictatorship had renamed. The parties were much smaller, much quieter, with fewer high-end types thanks to the nightly crypt of curfew. Certain clubs managed to stay open, as the military never chased down the homo erectus like they did in Argentina and Brazil. Maybe a complacent homosexuality didn't threaten their moral scruples. Maybe there were too many right-wing locas supporting the dictatorship. Or maybe the French perfume that wealthy gays wore merely covered up the stench of rotting bodies. Either way, the dictatorship's mortuary stink turned out to be just a teaser for AIDS, which would make its debut in the early eighties.

Of this short synopsis of liberty, the only thing left is the UNCTAD, the giant cement elephant that sheltered the military for years. Democracy later reclaimed its terraces and patios, though all the sculptures donated by Popular Unity artists are no longer there. The huge auditoriums and conference rooms, too, have been reclaimed, where they now host forums dedicated to homosexuality, AIDS, utopias, and tolerance.

There's only one photo left from that party, a bleached snapshot where the sissy faces reappear, exposed to the present at a distance. It's not a good photo, but their sexual militancy jumps out at the viewer. The receding years frame them, their mouths are extinguished laughter, echoes of gestures frozen in the flash of a final toast. Jokes, sneers, quips, and shade drip from their lips, ready to fall, ready to lace their kisses with irony. It's not a good photo, the image blurry, an unfocused haze that never stabilizes into memory. Maybe the photo is fuzzy because the stained tulle of AIDS shrouds almost every loca in a double disappearance. That shadow, it's a fragile cellophane bandage that wraps around la Pilola Alessandri's waist as she leans her faggot hips against the right side of the table. She purchased the epidemic in New York, the first one to bring it back, the genuine article, the latest, most exclusive gay trend in how to die. The hottest mortuary look, which made her drop pounds faster than any diet, leaving her as skinny and pale as the models in *Vogue*, as stretched and chic as an orchid's sigh. AIDS wrung out her body, and she died pressed and pleated, fashionable and stunning in the rarefied ranks of her miserly death.

It's not a good photo. No one knows if it's black and white, or if the color simply fled to warmer climates. No one knows if their blushes and the withered roses on the plastic tablecloth were slowly washed away by floods and rain while the photo hung from a nail in la Palma's shack of a home. It's hard to decode the chromatics, to imagine color into blouses speckled by frost each impoverished winter. Just humidity's yellow halo lending the photo some life. Moldy traces light the paper, spilling into a stain across la Palma's chest. They pierce her, pinning her like a butterfly in the AIDS cabinet of curiosities. She was caught in Brazil, after she'd sold her chicken stand at La Vega, when she couldn't bear the military any longer and decided to maraca her way to the sands of Ipanema. Why bother being a loca, if not to live out Carnaval and take life at a two-step? Besides, at thirty-nine pesos to the dollar, the Rio piñata hung within reach. The chance to be queen for a night, at the cost of your life. "And what of it," she said in the airport in her rich-girl pantomime. "You blow what you have, that's all."

AIDS was generous with la Palma, wallowing, loitering among the countless starving degenerates who wanted sex. You might say AIDS was handed to her on a platter, sliced and diced to death along Copacabana's molten aqueduct. La Palma sipped Kaposi's serum to the last drop, gorging herself on her own ending. Burning with fever, she'd head back to the beach, handing out the contagious party streamer to every street kid, delinquent, and leper she met in the shadow of its Black Orpheus. Hers was an AIDS drunk on threesomes and samba, and it swelled her up like a faded balloon, like a condom blown up by the wheeze of her pious asshole, the asshole that never stopped giving, echoing with tambourines and timbales in the passion of AIDS-wrought diarrhea. Like a big party, a samba class for dying sequined and scattered in the thrum of the favelas, in the pours of African perfume that soaked the dirt roads to black and washed over Avenida Atlântica, the street in Rio always willing to sin and be repaid in flesh for its delirious pleasures.

La Palma came back and died happy in her agony, stripped of her savings. She said goodbye listening to Ney Matogrosso's music, humming the saudade of her parting. "See you at the next party," she said sadly, gazing at the photo nailed to the wallboards of her misery. And right before she closed her eyes, she looked so young again, almost a blushing maid raising a glass and a fistful of bones that summer of 1973. She looked so beautiful in the photo's reflection, wrapped in la Pilola's white mink, so queenly in the halo of albino fur, that she told the Ghost, Hold on a sec, and held back Death's bony hand while she took one last look at herself, indulged her narcissus in furs for one final moment. Then she closed her lids and let herself go, floating away on a velvet memory.

It's a bad photo, the shot hastily taken because the locas couldn't stop fidgeting, almost all of them blurred by too many poses and their wild desire to leap into the future. Practically a last supper of queer apostles, where the only thing clearly rendered is the pyramid of bones on the table. It might be mistaken for a biblical frieze, a Holy Thursday watercolor caught in the vapors rising from the jug of wine that la Chumi holds like a Chilean goblet. She stuck herself right in the middle, standing in Christ's stead, everything but the altar lamps. The twenty-centimeter-high heels keeping la Chumi on her toes, showing off her travesti glamour. In la Pilola's black mink fur, she becomes a virginal native, who sighs delicately, the pelt slipping off the white slopes of her shoulders, an animal embrace warming her fragile heart. All muff, all rosebud gloved in the fur's branches. Like an old Hollywood photo in the haughty turn of her cheek for a kiss. Just a kiss, la Chumi seems to say to the camera. A single kiss from the flash so she's covered in sparkles, blinded by her own mirror. Her lying mirror, her false image of proletariat diva turning a loaf of bread and some tomatoes into breakfast for her family. She defended her whoring territory with a switchblade, ready to call anyone out who stepped on her corner of the sodomite beat. La Chumilou was tough, the other travestis said. You had to tread carefully if some new girl had lifted one of her clients. La Chumi was the favorite, the one they always wanted, the sole comfort of bored husbands who entushed themselves in the scent of a passionate fag. And so the AIDS hook chose her as bait for its miraculous catch. For skipping meals, for all those handjob handouts, for reaping what she sowed under the moon's silver coin. For being greedy, not checking to see if she had another condom in her purse. And there was so much money, so many bills—so many dollars this gringo was willing to pay. So much makeup, so many depilatory machines and jars of wax. So many dresses and new shoes so she could finally ditch her ugly old clogs. So many eggs, so much bread and pasta she could bring home. There were so many dreams stuck in that fistful of dollars. So many siblings whose hungry mouths haunted her night after night. Her mother whose mouth was full of rotten molars, who had no money for the dentist but couldn't sleep from the pain and so waited up for Chumilou until morning. There were so many debts, so many school enrollment fees, so much she needed to pay, because she wasn't ambitious like the other locas said she was. La Chumi made do with next to nothing, just a few thrift-store fineries, a frilly blouse and a skirt, a faded rag that her mother sewed a bit here, pulled something through there, gluing on sequins and lace to spruce up la Chumi's work uniform, saying be careful, don't get in bed with just anyone, don't forget the condoms, which she bought for la Chumi each week at the corner pharmacy, overcoming her shame. But that night la Chumi ran out, and the gringo was impatient, crazy to get inside her, waving that green fan of dollars. So la Chumi closed her eyes and reached out her hand to clutch the wad of bills. Her luck couldn't be so bad that this one time—if this one time in how many years she did it in the flesh—the shadow would snatch her. And so, without wanting to, la Chumi stepped through the disease's curtained portico and gingerly entered its slimy waters, reserving her one-way ticket on its sinister ferry. I was bound to get kidnapped someday, she kept saying. Besides, I've already lived so much—my twenty-five years have been so long that when death finds me, I'll consider it a vacation. Bury me dressed as a woman, please, in my work clothes, with my metallic clogs and black wig. In my red satin dress, which always brought me good luck. No jewels, I'm leaving my diamonds and emeralds to my mother, so she can fix her teeth. The ranch and summer houses are for my little brothers and sisters, who deserve a good future. And for my fairy travestis, I leave the fifty-room mansion the Sheik gave me as a gift. So the oldest girls can retire somewhere nice. No wailing, none of that funeral stuff, the scratchy floral wreaths bought at the last minute from the flower stand. Especially not those live-forevers, which never dry out, as if you'd never finish dying. A single withered orchid at most, laid across my breast and sprinkled with dew. With real candles, not the tacky electric ones. Lots of candles. Hundreds of candles covering the floor, every surface, under the stairs, shining on San Camilo Street, on Vivaceta and Maipú and in La Sota de Talca. As many candles as we used in the blackouts, as many candles as the disappeared. Tons of little flames flickering over the city's wet stitches. Like burning sequins for our rainy streets. Thousands of candles like pearls from an unthreaded necklace, like coins from a smashed piggy bank. So many, like sparkles ripped from a neckline, or sparks from a halo, lighting the path . . . I'll need their warm glow to make me look like I've simply fallen asleep. Just a bit rosy from Death's vampire kiss. Almost unreal in the trembling aura of candlelight, almost sublime, sunk beneath the glass. Let everyone say, Maybe Chumi is asleep, like Sleeping Beauty, like a serene and untouched virgin whose miracle death erased every scar. No traces of disease, no bruises, no pustules, no bags under her eyes. My makeup should be snow-white, even if you completely have to redo my face. Like Ingrid Bergman in *Anastasia* or La Betty Davis in *Jezebel*, almost a little girl who fell asleep waiting. And I hope it's right before sunrise, like returning home from the palace after dancing all night long. No funeral procession, no priests, no dreary sermons. No poor-little-fairy, forgive-him-Lord-and-let-him-pass-into-your-kingdom. None of that crying or fainting, no tragic goodbyes. I'm going having earned my keep, *que me voy bien pagá*, like a cabaret singer hitting her final note. No need to pray for me or bestow the kisses that not even love ever gave. Look, there I go, walking across the foam. Look at me one last time, jealous, since I'm not coming back. I'm lucky I won't. I can feel Death's damp silk gagging my eyes, and so you can say I was happy right up to the end. I'll take nothing with me, as I had nothing, and I lost even that.

La Chumilou died the day democracy arrived, and her meager retinue crossed paths with the crowds that marched down the Alameda celebrating the NO vote's victory. It wasn't easy to weave through the mass of young painted faces, people waving the rainbow flag, yelling, singing jubilantly, hugging the locas who walked behind la Chumi's hearse. And for a moment pain blurred with joy, with sorrow, with carnival. As if Death had stepped out of the hearse to dance a final round of cueca. As if you could still hear la Chumi's morbid voice when she found out they'd won the election. Tell democracy I say hello, she said. And it would seem that democracy personally returned the greeting, in the hundreds of shirtless kids who bent over the hearse, hopping onto its roof, hanging from its windows, spray-painting the whole vehicle with graffiti that said: BYE TIRANO. HASTA NEVER, PINOCHITO. DEATH TO THE JACKAL. And la Chumi's mother watched in horror as the hearse transformed into an allegorical vehicle, inside a rowdy swirl of people who kept it company for a number of blocks. Afterward the car returned to its march of mourning, to its pachyderm trot through the deserted streets toward the cemetery. Someone had stuck a flag, with its victorious rainbow, among the flower wreaths. A white flag streaked with color, which followed la Chumi all the way to her winter garden.

Maybe that photo from la Palma's party is all that's left from an era of social utopias, when the locas caught a glimpse of their future emancipation. They took part in that euphoria, interwoven among the masses. Whether to the right or the left of Allende, they banged on pots and pans and spoke out, slowly refining the stories they told in shy glimpses and stammering speeches, recounting these minority histories in pursuit of legality.

Almost no one from that photo is still alive. The pale yellow paper is a faded sun, an eviction served to these locas even as their skin brightens the daguerreotype. Flies' dirty feet have spotted their cheeks with moles, as if anticipating sarcoma's makeover. All the faces mottled by that pustulous rain. All their laughs perched on the photo's balcony—each one a handkerchief waved from an invisible prow. Before the millennial ship docks at 2000, before, even, the legalization of homosexuality in Chile, before the nineties gay militancy brought homosexuals together. Before masculine fashion imposed itself like the uniform of some redeeming army—before neoliberalism, disguised as democracy, gave us permission to breed. Long before these perks, the photo of the locas at the New Year's party registers like something glimmering in an underwater world. Their laughter's crystalline obscenity is still subversive, turning upside down any assumptions about gender. The crumpled photo still measures the distance between then and now, the years of dictatorship that forced masculinity into our mannerisms. The homosexual's demise and metamorphosis at the end of the century can be confirmed; locas kaposied by AIDS, but decimated first and foremost by an imported model of being gay, so fashionable, so penetrative in its angling for power, the masculine homosexual supernova. In the photo the locas wave the century goodbye, their tattered plumage still lopsided, still folksy in their illegal ways. It almost looks like an archaic frieze from an era before the gay patriarch's meddling had left its mark. From an era before the plague spread to native lands, recolonizing via bodily fluids. The photo shows a gleaming carousel, the whirling chirps of laughter so young, so adolescent in their distorted hoarding of what the world might hold. A whole other corpus determined their tribal rituals. Other deliriums baroquely enriched discussions about Latin American homosexualities. The faggoted Chilean still stitched herself a future, dreaming of her emancipation alongside other social causes. The invention of "Mister Gay," or "the homosexual man," had a narcissistic potency that didn't fit inside the malnourished frame of the locas' mirrors. Those bodies, those muscles, those biceps that foreign magazines advertised to us, were a first-world Olympus, an educated gym class, a bodybuilding culture obsessed with its own reflection. This new territory for the old blond ideal caught on fast among the social-climbing malinches, those well-traveled queens who got the model straight from New York and carried it back to this far corner of the world. And tucked into this Superman mold, right against the sterile gauze of its white skin—so hygienic, so perfumed in capitalist charm, so far from the dark leather of our geography—in this Apollo, in his smooth-cheeked marble, the syndrome found shelter and showed up on our shores like some traveler, like a tourist who was just passing through Chile until our blood's sweet wine made him stay.

The fact that la Palma, la Pilola Alessandri, and la Chumilou all met the same fate speaks to AIDS as a public courier, free of social bias. The contagious hand flaunts a deadly generosity in its silent redistribution. It seems to say: There's enough to go around, no need to push. I won't run out, don't worry. Until they find a cure, there's passion and torment for all.

Maybe small histories and grand epics never run in parallel, with minority destinies scorched by a market always on the prowl for defectors. Any fissures on the hypercontrolled modernist map are detected and patched with the same cement—the same mix of cadavers and dreams—that lies beneath the neoliberal pyramid's scaffolding. Maybe that final glint in la Palma's, la Pilola's, and la Chumilou's eyes was a wish, or really three wishes, all stuck waiting for the furs to appear. Because no one ever knew where those fabulous coats ended up that evening. They evaporated into the summer night, like a stolen dream, which picks up again but further on, beyond nostalgia—somewhere in the seropositive winters of those locas, when the plague's snowy cotton frosted over their feet.

THE DEATH OF MADONNA

The mystery struck her down first. These days almost every travesti who lives on San Camilo Street is infected, but the clients keep coming, seem to like it even better, since they fuck without condoms.

We just knew her as Madonna, though that wasn't always her name. But it was love at first sight when she saw that gringa singing on TV, practically went crazy trying to imitate her, copying every gesture, her laugh, the way she moved. La Madonna was from Temuco, she had a real Mapuche look to her, so we used to tease her, calling her Moccasin Madonna, Suckatash Madonna, Our Lady of the Backwaters. She didn't mind though, even if that's why she dyed her hair blonde, real blonde, practically white. But the mystery had already done its damage by then. When she bleached her roots with that hydrogen peroxide her hairs came out with the brush, fell from her head in ugly clumps. So we called her mangy bitch for a while, but she never did want to wear a wig. Not even the gorgeous platinum one we gave her for Christmas, which wasn't cheap, all the travestis had chipped in to buy it downtown with the loose change we'd added up, coin by coin, for months. Just so the girl could start working again and cheer up a bit. But she was too proud—she thanked us with tears in her eyes, clutching the wig to her heart as she explained that a true star couldn't accept these sorts of gifts, even from her fans.

Before the mystery, that hussy had such nice hair, she'd wash it every day and sit on the stoop, combing out knots in the sun. We were always telling her, get inside, girl, the police will drive by any minute, but she always ignored us, our patter no more bother than the rain. She never was afraid of the cops. She'd stop them all high-and-mighty, shouting that she was an artist and not a murderer like them. Then they'd thrash her hard, beating her until she collapsed on the pavement, though never enough to make her shut up, she'd keep howling until their van disappeared. They left her looking like bruised quince, all black and blue down her spine, her kidneys, her face. Huge welts no powder could cover up. But she just laughed. They hit me because they love me, she'd say, with those teeth that dropped like pearls out of her mouth, one after another. Later on she didn't like to laugh anymore, switched to drinking, she'd gulp down anything and finish her night on the pavement just the same, so drunk it hurt to see her.

Without hair or teeth, she was no longer the same Madonna who made us laugh when work was slow. We'd spend our nights sitting in the doorway, cold as shit, cracking jokes. And she'd always be copying Madonna in her tiny skirt, which was actually a pullover that was too long for her. A ribbed turtleneck, wool with sparkly threads, the kind of thing you'd find at a thrift shop. She'd cinched it with a belt and, voilà, a miniskirt. A real queen of creativity, always turning some rag into a dress.

Of course once she got her implants she switched to plunging necklines. The clients would go crazy inside their cars when she pushed her tits up against the glass. And for a split second it seemed like the real Madonna had appeared before them, saying: Míster, lovmi plís.

She knew the words to every song but had no idea what they meant. She parroted the sounds and phrases, hauling in whatever got caught in the torn net of her alphabet. Not that she really needed to know what the blondie was really trying to say. Her oyster mouth modulated every tuyú, each miplís, all the remember lovmis. If you closed your eyes, she was Madonna, and it wasn't just a healthy dose of imagination helping us envision her Mapuche twin so clearly. Because thousands of clippings of the star papered Madonna's room. Thousands of pieces of her heavenly body formed the loca's private constellations. An entire world of newsprint and glossy magazine pages hiding the cracks in the wall, covering with winks and Marilyn Monroe kisses the mildew stains, the bloody fingerprints wiped on the walls, the traces of that violent rogue concealed by the blurry A-listers who orbited the singer. And so a thousand Madonnas hovered around a single light caked with dead bugs that yellowed the room, variations on the same infinite image in every shape, in every size, at every age—a star continually resurrected in the plush love of a besotted loca. Right until the end, when she could no longer get up, when AIDS knocked her flat on her filthy mattress. Her dying wish was simply to listen to a Madonna cassette and hold a photo of the singer across her heart.

It must have been the late eighties, or around then, when corporeal performance was blowing up the Chilean art world. When a vulnerable body could still speak to the dictatorship's horrors. Maybe there was so much barbed wire twisted around our cultural framework that no one predicted anything like *Gone with AIDS*, or could have imagined the way its metaphor would coagulate in some of the participants from San Camilo. A street that was home to travesti lives and the kind of sex work that was already beginning to disappear from Santiago.

The art action was staged in their honor, an homage that unfolded a starry night sky on the dirty cement. A Broadway parody drawn in sodomy, scratched into Latin American mud.

The stars, some of them filled in and others left as outlines, underscored the title's poetics. Spotlights and movie cameras turned it into a Hollywood-style production, the travestis looking more beautiful than ever, all dolled up for the premiere, posing for the independent media, debuting the silicone fresh in their tits. The camera flashes blinding the neighborhood. And the eyes of the whole cultural resistance under dictatorship—the politicians, artists, intellectuals, photographers, and filmmakers—bulging like frogs' at the sight of the Yeguas del Apocalipsis, who were raining stars over the main drag of travesti sex.

For one night only, the neighborhood girls dreamed under the tropical bloom of a movie set and cast themselves in Chinese theater. A mini Malibu reflected in whatever the third world had on hand, the diva's universe a street of broken mirrors, the stars like shards of glass forming a mirage that drew out the city's anal whores and streetwalking masquerade.

And no one was more photographed than Madonna. Not for being pretty—more for her lewd, mischievous gestures. For the sappy halo that crowned her pouts, her mutant body that contorted generously to meet every greedy photographer's flash.

She was the only one who believed it all, pressing her thick hands into the wet cement. The only one who afterward let a young videographer keep recording her. The only one who posed nude for the woman's camera under the shower. Bare as the day God chucked her into the world, but hiding her shameful member between her cheeks. The travesti's Chinese lock, which pretends to be a vagina by tucking back the whole cluster. A DIY surgery that's convincing at first, passing for the feminine modesty of thighs squeezed tightly shut. But, after a while, under so much scrutiny, with all that heat, with that warm narcissus propped at the doors of self-conception, the trick springs free like a rubber band, a surprise pendulum that bursts through her virginal pose, the goddess's surgical fraud caught forever on tape.

Several years went by, the political changes finally came, and democracy organized the first official exhibition of censored art. The National Museum of Fine Arts and its reinstated director, Nemesio Antúnez, gave the thumbs-up for *Museo Abierto*, a huge show that covered every genre of visual art, including photography, video, and performance.

They set up one of the galleries just to screen the films, and on opening day an impressive number of visitors crowded into these spaces of newfound creative liberty. Since the whole point of the exhibition was that it was uncensored, Our Virgin of San Camilo had slipped right through in *Casa particular*, a film that Gloria Camiruaga had made on the travesti streets with the help of the Yeguas. But at noon, that hour when schoolchildren visit museums, bringing with them their fidgeting ruckus, during whatever recess or lunch that education sets aside for art, a squadron of scouts planted themselves in the video gallery along with their chaperone, Daniel Boone, who hoped to civilize their savage ways. And after watching reel after reel of dreary testimonials about torture, overly conceptual music videos, and boring short films by video artists who wished they were directors in Hollywood, and after the kiddos, forced into appreciating the arts, began to feel the heavy sweet weight of sleep. Smack in the middle of this boring field trip the screen lit up with la Madonna's naked body and the little whelps burst into applause, especially the ones who were a little bigger than the others. Ecological scout leader Boone groped for his glasses and caught the camera panning across the loca's hairless body: her native features, her Hellenic shoulders pulled down so that she's shyly posing like a nymph, her small nipples bunched up as her arms push them together. And those arms! And the camera gliding over her smooth stomach like a toboggan. And everyone panting, the kiddos grabbing their green winkles. The oldest among them gasping with excitement as the camera slides down the torso. Each of their camping shorts pitching a tent at the very moment that the screen's gaze lands squarely in pubic pastures. Everyone silent, clenched in silence, eyes glued as the camera probed that dark forest, that fake pleat, that fissure Madonna had made by holding her breath and squeezing her prostate between her glutes, feigning a demure Venus for the art connoisseurs, for the camera prying between her legs. Then the slinky slips and an intractable phallus spills onto the screen, practically hitting the brigade leader in the face. And for a moment there's just kiddos laughing and clapping, just surprise when the dam breaks and Madonna's genitals rush in, a scream in Morse code that shocks the room. Just chaotic fun as the gallery fills with even more student visitors grabbing playfully at each other, touching themselves, watching the rapid metamorphosis on a loop, the film's scene on tireless repeat. Just an emergency for the museum employees trying to pull the tape. For the scout leader shouting at them to stop this obscenity, this outrage that has no name, didn't they think about the minors, who were busy clutching their stomachs laughing. Again and again her member bursts the illusion, again and again Madonna reveals the trick, her travesti cock that swings like the clapper of a bell, alerting the whole museum as the secretaries and assistants sprint toward the room, causing so much mayhem, so much shouting from the teachers and scout leader tugging at his whistle, clamoring for them to cut the nastiness, this isn't art, this is pornography, one hundred percent libertine muck dragging the democracy down. How in the world had the esteemed Señor Nemesio Antúnez allowed such a show to take place? And why hadn't someone brought him down here already, so he could take some responsibility for this botched horror? Because only he could order the film strip to be pulled. Then Nemesio—who'd never seen the video—arrived and, after meeting Madonna and her playful marionette, gave orders to cut the tape. And explained with his sincerest apologies that in this case censorship did apply.

Maybe la Madonna never heard about these difficulties, which earned the director an earful straight from the president's mouth. Maybe she never knew about the gray hairs Nemesio sprouted as he was heckled by journalists who asked, Can you explain why you are censoring art in a democracy? Maybe she didn't know her naive performance would lead to other artists being kicked out of the show. Or know about the right-wing critics, who were always only too happy to point out the young democracy's moral slips and spills. La Madonna never knew a thing, she was too far away from all that cultural production, sewing lace onto a chemise to wow her anonymous visitors. She'd spend her afternoons gluing sequins to a sheer hem to round out her hips. Testing out her creations whenever she drifted to the newspaper stand on the corner to buy a single cigarette. That was where she saw the headline that Madonna was on tour in Latin America. She knew the singer would appear in a flock of Boeings that would be carrying her superstar production. She couldn't talk about anything else after that. We're going to be friends, she'd say, one look at me and she'll see we were made for each other. Maybe we'll even do a show together—that is, if she doesn't want to use me as her double for interviews. Because there are so many things she has to do exhausted, poor thing. All the tours and airplanes, all the men chasing her backstage. I'd be her best friend, her confidante, her right hand—the only person who can get her to fall asleep without taking pills. Just lemon balm tea and a warm bath with eucalyptus, massaging her feet as I tell her my life story until we end up snoring together in her huge black satin bed.

Maybe if Madonna had gotten wind of these dreams, if she'd received even one of her fan letters, she'd have extended her tour to our far end of the world. But her Boeings never did make it across the cordillera, the diva got only as far as Buenos Aires, where her show was so scandalous she gave our Catholic-Andean morals a rash. And that led to her show being canceled in Chile. The authorities claimed that there wasn't any censorship, but "simply a lack of commercial sponsors for Madonna in our country." So everyone knew that, behind the scenes, the white glove of morality had done its dirty work, shooing the goddess of sex and her attendants back to the first world.

The Virgin of San Camilo never recovered from the pain of her dashed hopes, and the AIDS shadow darkened along with the bags under her eyes, snuffing her out with failure after failure. From that moment on, her sparse albino hair began to molt in a snowfall of feathers that dusted the sidewalk along her cruising routes, where she'd stop in front of a car, all harsh in her stilettos, her lipstick smeared, wiggling her loose teeth with her tongue as she leaned into the window to ask, Míster, yu lovmi?

And bringing the show to an end, she closed her eyes, her mascara like a heavy curtain falling to thunderous applause. The final dance number cut short. Her breathing shallow and rough, the motor inside her chest is a sports car stuck on the French Riviera. Her mouth is half-open, its pink tinge fading in the plumage of decline, her lips are a kiss that flies past the lens that never caught this other Madonna, a last kiss caressing a peachy cheek that then falls against her shoulder, skin flecked with a sheen of sweat like stars constellating her last night on earth. Her insides are unraveling, her ravaged body is now just a shadow under her miniskirt, an unlucky break after the diva's contextured elasticity. She's without a partner for this last dance, spinning alone beyond where our eyes can see, waving goodbye at the airport, burned by the camera flashes, the photographs deifying her like some infinitely reproducible factory doll. No one can reach her as she runs down the staircase at the stroke of midnight, her high heels echoing on the silver steps. Fleeing the farce of celebrity, alienated from Monroe and from her own self, how ironic, that original movie poster where two Madonnas return to the old dirty neighborhood. Maybe the only place they could find each other, humming a song, sharing a pack of gum, and swapping secrets about the best way to dye their hair.

LETTER TO LIZ TAYLOR

(OR, EGYPTIAN EMERALDS FOR AZT)

And so, dear Liz, without knowing if the soft calypso of your eyes will ever read this letter.

What's worse—and knowing how busy you are—I'm adding myself to your grand tally, to the infected multitudes who write to ask you for a little something. Maybe an autograph, a lock of your hair, the lace from your slip—I don't know, any trifle that lets them die knowing you received their message. But the thing is, I don't want to die, or receive a printed autograph, or even a photo of you and Montgomery Clift in Raintree County. *Nothing like that, just an emerald from the crown you wore in that Cleopatra film, which they say was real. So genuine that a single gem could add years to my life, on pure AZT.*

I don't mean to pressure you with my morbid crocodildo tears or rob you of something so dear. Think of me as freeing you from these gems that have been cursed by pharaohs and that always bring bad luck in the end, luring thieves to ransack your house. And I'm not joking either, you remember what happened to Sharon Tate, nothing funny about that. Not to mention the wisps of gossip, the vipers who murmur that your jewels must be swimming in your wrinkles. How you've got no neck left for new baubles. How a queen shouldn't be flashy, how at your age such sparkling rubies clash with your cellulite. How, in short, with so many hungry, you flit from jewel to jewel, and even Julio Iglesias went cross-eyed from so much glare. How the checks you write for AIDS—which you sign so fervently—end up clutched by the same fingers that traffic the plague. And, listen to this, they say that your piety is just for show, entirely promotional, you see, like the campaign's symbol, the little red ribbon that for all the poor faggots is actually plastic and made in Taiwan. And the rich with theirs in rubies and gold, looking more like a noose, that deadly necktie. A way of signaling who won the prize—you know how people are, fighting over anything. They've even said you're sick with it, too, which explains the weight loss. It's enough to glance at photos from a few years ago, when there wasn't a single dress you fit in. And now so much love for the leper homosexuals. So much affection for Jackson, our pop music Christ, who sings, "Suffer the little children to come to me." How funny, this little enthusiasm of yours. So much love for the fags, just like Liza Minnelli, Barbra Streisand, and María Félix. All these stars who suckle locas like cuddly puppies. As if faggots were another kind of charming ornament. As if they were the Jewel of the Nile or the final gleam of a submerged Atlantis. How funny, and yet—for the lesbians, not a peep. When really, the lesbians say, it should be the other way around. First sisterly solidarity, then the locas. There's even a word in New York for the rich and famous who run all over town with their hairstylists and couturiers.

. . . I think it's all trash, Liz, they're just jealous. Besides, us fairies, we have the heart of a star and a soul of platinum, which is why I feel so close to you. Which is why you'll understand the reason I'm asking you this favor. If it's what you want, if it isn't too much trouble. I would be terminally in your debt. Remember, a tiny emerald, only a few carats, small enough that you barely notice when they take it out of the crown. Plus you have those turquoises to look at, which outshine every other sparkle. I live in Chile, mail it to me at the return address. I don't think you've ever been to this country. They say there's lots of money here, but you wouldn't know it, not from the look of things.

Your admirer, para siempre.

THE MILLION NAMES OF MARÍA CHAMELEON

The gay zoo—like clouds lacquered in blushes, mannerisms, and contempt—seems to be in constant flight from its own identity. No single name or exact geography to define their desires, their passions, their furtive wanderings through the night's subterranean agenda, where they all casually bump into each other, never failing when they say hello to make up new badges and nicknames that allude to small cruelties, funny anecdotes, and zoomorphic caricatures. A collection of shorthands that hide the baptismal roster, the father's mark consecrated in his butch offspring, that Luis Jr. branded on him for life. Never asking, never understanding, never knowing if Alberto, Arturo, or Pedro would suit his delicate fag of a son, who's stuck with this prostate of a name until he dies. That's why he can't stand the parental tattoo, that call, that Luchito, that little handicapped Hernancito, which for homosexuals means only more taunting and disdain.

So, the name question can't be fixed simply by swapping out Carlos for Carla. There's a huge baroque allegory that enfeathers, enlivens, traverses, disguises, dramatizes, or punishes identity through a nickname—the whole thing like some loony bin folk legend, plucking pseudonyms out of cinema's starry firmament. The pubescent maids and beloved heroines, the worshipped divas, but also the evil stepmothers and hooker harpies. Names, adjectives, and nouns that continually rebaptize depending on the looks, mood, niceness, bitchiness, or boredom of a sodomite clan always willing to reroute the party, to tease out a name's semiotics to exhaustion.

Nobody's spared, especially not the sisters with AIDS, who are cataloged on a parallel list requiring triple inventiveness to keep up humor's remedy, the perpetually cheerful attitude, the gags on the fly so the virus can't fade her live-forever smile. No single nickname sticks around long enough to tattoo her dying face, since there are a thousand names that can shatter the sanctimony of a clinic appointment. Ten thousand ways to make a seropositive friend laugh, so that depression doesn't weaken her immune system. A million tiny distractions to get her laughing at herself, mocking her own drama. Starting with the name.

The poetics of the gay nickname generally goes further than just identifying someone: the name disfigures, smears any features recorded in bureaucratic registers. The name doesn't encompass a single way of being, it's closer to a profile that briefly includes many, the hundreds who pass at some time through the same epithet.

The list of nicknames includes what might be a prickly humor, an acid ascertainment of those imperfections and irregularities our bodies must painfully endure—sometimes a limp, or hemiplegia, those many subtle flaws that become so hard to conceal, adding insult to the real injury. But in this case the nickname lightens the load, illuminating with little altar lamps a defect that only hurts more for trying to hide it. A nickname turns a hairy mole into a velvet dune. That fucked-up hump? An odalisque Sahara. Those myopic eyes? A dreamy geisha. That peewee dwarfism? A demure Lilliputian. That hatchet nose? A glacier of breath. That calamitous obesity? A white and pink cloud à la Rubens. That bald spot covered by a part drawn practically at the ear? A cranial shine of good luck. Those elephant ears? A pair of flamenco fans. That mailbox mouth? A stormy, absorbing kiss. In short, there's always a metaphor that, in ridiculing, beautifies the flaw, making it unique, one's own. A nickname that hurts at first but later makes even the girl herself laugh. What starts as overexposure to a shame constantly yelled and named and pointed out turns into a ghetto rebaptism that camouflages the real name. A reconversion where caricature becomes a sign of affection.

And there are loads of ways to name yourself. For the standard feminine variation, just add an "a" to the tail of Mario, and you get "Simply María." Or choose the maternal complicity of family: the mamas, godmamas, grandmamas, cousin-mamas, sister-mamas, mamitas, etc. Or any of those countryish characters who turn up in folklore—the innocence of a Carmela, or Chela, or Rosa, or Maiga, etc. The most sophisticated can take on the Remember Me Hollywood-esque of la Garbo, la Dietrich, la Monroe, la West. But, here in Latin America, our celluloid memory has consecrated its own virgins: la Sara Montiel, la María Félix, la Lola Flores, la Carmen Miranda. No one knows why locas adore these grandes dames so much, who recede further each decade into the sepia of their photos. No one knows, but the thousands of travestis who copy them have homosexualized these names, imitated their gestures and bullfighter gazes. Every faggot has a Félix inside him, or a Montiel, and he brings her out when the streetlights turn on, when the moon skins itself on the clouds.

The list keeps growing—as long as fashion insists on stars with a bit of class and homo flair, as long as a stock of names helps camouflage the family signage, as long as humor helps ease the retroviral burden. So here are a few, solely and exclusively for show, plucked from the prickly fields of pansy culture.

La Pit of Despair
La Walkout
La Once Again
La Just Because
La Not Today Satan
La Silicone María
La Triple-Threat María
La Windbreaker
La Sour Puss
La Suckerpunch María
La Maripepa
La Nefer-titi

La Lola Flores
La Sara Montiel
La Carmen Sevilla
La Carmen Miranda
La María Félix
La Fabiola of Luján
Our Lady of the Crazy Purse
Our Lady of the Empanada
Our Lady of the Piano
Our Lady of the Bun
La Tail on the Corner
La Multipurpose
La Mover and Shaker
La Modern Woman
La Handbrake
La Paramour
La Kermit the Frog
La Joint
La Barefoot Hippie
La Bare
La Posh
La Hoity-Toity
La French Pout
La Chumilou
La Trolleybus
La Scandalous Sandra
La False Hope
La Lola Jackknife
La No Way
La Sell Your Soul
La Coupon Queen
La No Guarantees
La Petronila Perestroika
La Stiletto Ass
La Seven Asses
La Stick It Up Yours
La Wheezy Ass
La Daphne Duck

La Wendy
La There She Comes
La There She Goes
La Rosie the Riveting
La Bada Bim Bada Bum
La Cucu
La Indy Cola
La Coca-Cola
La Bootycall
La Lola
La Rose
La Denise
La Susi
La Pupi
La Mimi
La Bambi
La Tete
La Toto
La Nene
La Lulu
La Chica Almodóvar
La Bottle Popper
La Blowjob Minister
La Million-Dollar Suck
La Blender
La Multimatic
La Adorable
La Motorbike
Our Lady Hamburger Helper
La Clinic Queen
La All Good
La Ninja
La Karate Kid
La Here I Come
La Naughty Nurse
La Baby Teeth
La Ass-assin
La Headscissor

La Mystery María
La Deficient María
La Risky María
La Aspirin María
La Sarcoma María
La AZT María
La Kool-AIDS
La Worry Warts
La Narci-cyst
La Pay-to-Play
La Forget-Me-Not
La Yes We Can
La Voilà AIDS
La Voilà Kaposi
La AIDS Frappé
La AIDS on the Rocks
La Band-AIDS
La Bugs Bonnie
La Lynne-phoma
La Gone with the Wind

REGINE, QUEEN OF MONKEY ALUMINUMS

And seeing how the plague is a firefly let loose in Santiago's slums, a dangerous North Star that replaces the alleyways' sunken streetlamps. Feeble gray light that all but hides the squalor of rags, cardboard, and rotting fruit on the pavement where la Regine is cruising in stilettos. The loca who stumbles half-drunk, half-dizzy from the AZT that's so hard to get hold of. But it always arrives somehow, contraband, or gotten half-price through some witchy bit of business. Sacred AZT, the gas for making life's wild party on the fourth floor last just a little longer. Regine's palace, where the show has always already started, the neon Monkey Aluminums sign illuminating the crowd bright red. Like some fifties movie where there's always an open window and a flickering promo that interrupts the kissing and casts the caresses in fluorescent light. Or, at least, advertises that every fondle has a price. And though the tenement shivers in every earthquake, and the walls that keep it propped up are spattered in urine, la Regine lives out what's left of her stigma *como si fuera esta noche la última vez*. As if at any moment the fifties movie might end with the girl waving goodbye at her window. And the only thing left of her story will be the neon Monkey Aluminums sign twitching on the screen.

Everyone in Mapocho knows and loves Regine's daily walk, when, shopping bag in hand, she crosses the road to snake between the stalls at La Vega. She's barely left the house but she's already sweaty, just like the shirtless workmen who call out to her: Regine, I still need to get my fill today! Regine, tonight's just for you! Oh, Regine, don't ever die, as she cups her fruit with her seashell hands, laughing and chitchatting with women whose tits are as huge as melons, who tell her: You're so skinny these days, Regine. What's that diet you're on? Look, you don't even have a butt anymore. Take these oranges, make yourself some juice and rest up. Don't let them give it to you so hard, men can never get enough. But Regine knows it's not a diet, and not men either—she herself is disappearing with every laugh, every tease she answers puckering and flirty as she bites into a peach. She is what's fading, like the red in the cherries she hangs from her ears. She's evaporating, mingling with the smells of sweet vanilla and the oregano she bought so she can make that pizza her man likes so much.

And Regine reigns over the fish and seafood market, too, which shimmers beneath her siren travesti charm. What will it be today, princess? the men ask with their hands covered in scales. Don't you want this beautiful orange crab? Look how juicy it is. Don't you want some mussels for your hangover? Or some pink barnacles for our Mona Lisa after yesterday's spanking at Monkey Aluminums? When music from the fourth-floor window could be heard late into the night. Palmenia Pizarro singing that cruel little waltz of hers, *En vano quieres matar mi orgullo. No has visto ni verás llanto en mis ojos*, Regine would murmur, clinging to her soldier, singing slowly so she can blow the lyrics into the swarthy ear of her buzzcut who they say is always at half-mast. *Y dicen que le hace pero no le hace, tan chiquitita y quiere casarse* with the loca who keeps him neat as a button. He's never had such clean white underwear laid out for him, not even by his own mother. Pure bleach and elbow grease so that he doesn't smell like sweaty feet anymore, the kid who now looks so pretty and smells so sweet when the regiment gives him a day off. When he takes Regine out for ice cream on those suffocatingly hot afternoons in La Vega.

He was the only one who stayed with her after the dictatorship ended. The only skinny grunt who Regine baptized as her official lover after doing roll call for the whole troop, for the rows of conscripts who entered her ass at a quick march. And who left having brushed up against their own burial flag.

Truckloads of men unloaded their powder there, combusting inside the Monkey Aluminums palace. There was always enough to go around—a midnight snack of ass stew for the burning troops. At all hours, after dinner or at the crack of dawn, when curfew was a bell jar over the city, until some scream cracked that bell and bullets rained down on the people who lived there. A scream that sullied the glass with a spatter of blood. Then the light from the fourth-floor window would be the only beacon for patrols tired of beating repression's music into the city's inhabitants with their nightsticks. That's when the patrol's commanding lieutenant would send one of his grunts over to Regine's place to ask if she could take them in, if the boys could rest there a little while, they'd bring a bottle of pisco and Regine wouldn't have to pay them any mind. But Regine minded them anyway. And out of nowhere she'd whip up a soup for the soldiers, something to stick to the bones, as she liked to say. With lots of onion and garlic, to get them each good and hard. Afterward they'd all file out to the locas' rooms. All except Sergio, that southern buzzcut who was as black as bull kelp. That soldier who played hard to get, saying he was tired, that he wanted to sleep, that he'd prefer to just sit on the stairs, teeth chattering, cold as shit, rather than ream a faggot.

He was the only one who never drank any pisco but smoked and smoked furiously, like he was chewing smoke, filling the whole floor with smoke to blot out the erotic scenes splayed out across Regine's couches. Like he didn't want to look, like if he smoked enough he could cover up sodomy's Sistine Chapel. Like he wanted to avoid being tempted by the rosy-cheeked asses that were swallowing those bayonets. Because Sergio never wanted to be a soldier, he hated the military and had been forced to enlist. Maybe that was why, repeating again and again that he was tired, would they please just leave him alone, the locas running their hands over him, saying, Why so sad? What's wrong? How 'bout a suck? They wouldn't leave him in peace, following him everywhere, wiggling their behinds until Regine snapped at them to stop dicking around. If he doesn't want to, he doesn't want to, don't be stupid. Tons of buzzcuts to gloat over and all you can do is annoy this poor kid. Not so poor, replied Sergio, turning to face her. But I have a conscience. And what is that, honey? La Regine, hands on her hips, her open silk robe revealing a flat nipple. I have feelings. But this is the house of feelings, love. You don't understand. And what should I understand, huh? The things that are going on. What things? Everything looks good to me. I'm all good. You don't think I look fabulous? Regine kneaded her shaved nipple. I meant other things. What things, huh, tell me, let's see. Sergio's voice caught and he couldn't answer, dodging Regine's sharp look. Tell me, huh, what're you afraid of? What's wrong. You can trust me, I'm silent as the grave. Come, she said, dragging Sergio over to the window where the sign's neon light turned the sill red. Santiago had disappeared into a sea of black tar. In the distance, glowing bonfires outed the night's protests. Barking dogs, gunshots, and explosions broke through the heavy leaden air. Can't you see what's going on? asked Sergio, nodding toward the horizon that couldn't sleep, kept up by gunfire's rhythms. It's a pretty song, said Regine, sounding sad. We could dance. But I'm not wearing heels, and I only dance in heels. Wait here a minute, I'll be right back. And right as she disappeared, a bombing cut the electricity, turning everything dark. The locas in the house shouted, Viva Chile! knotting hotly around the male protectors of the fatherland. Stay calm, stay calm, yelled the lieutenant, groping a young loca's smooth backside. Oh lieutenant, the terrorists, who never let us fu . . . sorry, live in peace.

The laughter fading, Sergio looked out again at the city, more impenetrable than ever in the swamp of the blackout. The window was no longer glowing, and the monkey's unlit neon skeleton was like a cutout pasted on a tragic sky. The wail of an ambulance made him jump just as he glimpsed a yellowy brightness coming down the hall. Regine, haloed in candlelight and dolled up, wearing black lace and high heels. Now we can dance, she murmured softly in his ear, whisking the tip of her tongue along those waxy folds. Sergio let her lick all around his hearing so he wouldn't have to listen to the powder keg drums. He let that suction block out the screams of women who grabbed onto the men he smacked with his gun as he dragged them out to the trucks. And so he let himself, too, be dragged, in Regine's effervescent slobber, so he didn't have to listen to the nylon rip of women's nightshirts as he separated them from their families. Now, the tip of her tongue ran over his sideburns and a hand was warming his manly clutch. He pulled it back abruptly but let Regine's tongue tickle his cheek, because it was like the tongue of a dog who licks the night's wounds, its giant abyss of living cadavers, licking his hands that were stiff from holding a gun. That warm tongue was a wet rag cradling the chin's tense muscles. It was a domesticated animal softening marble cheekbones right where a tear snakes down. A single drop that broke free from his tight heart. A tiny globe that makes everything blurry and traces slowly down his cheek to a tongue that slurps it up. As if—not speaking, not saying anything, not making a single sound—Regine was sipping his pain, her chatterbox tongue tracing the lines of Sergio's sad face. Like a paintbrush she traced his mouth, slashed by bitterness. His tight mouth, which he let be painted by that saliva bird. Her salty paintbrush that kissed his eyes and his forehead. And when Sergio was calmer, Regine peeled herself from his body, his whole face wet, avoiding his pupils, which kept shining through the blackness. That's all right, she said, after a moment, to signal that it was over. Now we talk.

No one knew what Sergio and Regine talked about that night, but they were always together after that. The patrols kept stopping by Monkey Aluminums to relax and wind down, until morning found them stark naked, lassoed by sheets runny with sweat and in the arms of a loca. Dawn's pale light reached through the windows, vanishing the orgy's petals. Everywhere glasses only half-drunk and cigarette butts. Everywhere parts of bodies scattered in sodomite disarray. An arm wrapped around a stomach, a leg tangled in oblivion. A brown torso with a loca's drool pooling on the chest. A buttock or two peeping out from the draped sheets, dripping with the fluids of the proletariat. An open hand that let go of the machine gun to grab something and froze like that, its empty gesture hollow and dead. Pairs of legs braided together, pressed into ass-fucking's hairy sandpaper mambo. Just like that, parts of bodies or cadavers stuck to the canvas of wrinkled sheets. Cadavers wearing lipstick and curled around their executioners. Still panting, still stretching out a hand to grab the flaccid faucet of the ejaculated war. Still alive, unfinished, crumbled somewhere beyond the window, floating in the city's tubercular haze that only the protests' gray smoke could clear.

So they were just playing dead, packages of skin squeezed dry in fits of orgasm. Limbs in repose that would jump up at the first ray of sunlight, disoriented, asking what time it was. Searching for their uniforms, the camouflage shirts and pants mixed with panties and high heels, a blonde wig crowning the rifle. They'd wake up emptying out the helmets that had been used as ashtrays. The rough cotton briefs the fatherland supplied them with tossed here and there and by the window. They'd fight over which pair was whose, figure it out by each of the boy's coloring. There was a redhead from the north, a Mapuche from the Araucanía, an albino with crimson eyes who could never find his eyeglasses and ran through the rooms twirling his huge flopping baton. In the chaos the lieutenant would ask where Sergio was. He's sleeping in the truck, they'd say. In the truck? Yes, just downstairs, right there in the truck, Regine would reply, opening her legs so that some wet-behind-the-ears beanpole could pull out. But you and Sergio . . . ? Sergio and I are friends. Nothing else. Don't you want some breakfast? And Regine would go into the kitchen to put the kettle on, leaving the lieutenant's question hanging.

Only long after the dictatorship ended did the lieutenant and his troops begin to understand Sergio and Regine's platonic love for each other. When diarrhea's cramps and cold sweats showed them the positive side of the epidemic. Madame Regine was already underground by then, planted like a fruit tree, and the entire La Vega neighborhood paid their respects on the silvery day of her funeral. The stalls were empty that afternoon, and when the pallbearers lowered the casket, petals fell like snow from the fourth-floor window. La Regine was so heavy, she'd swelled up, the poor thing, said the old ladies, we had to patch the cracks in the box so she wouldn't drip. But she dripped just the same, dirty tears that stained the stairs and the street for a long time. Purplish marks that the neighbors surrounded with candles as if they were miraculous shadows. Sergio was never seen again, he'd stayed by her side until that last day, when Regine told everyone to leave them alone for an hour. The locas glued themselves to the door, trying to listen from the outside, but no luck. Not a sigh or a noise. Not even the bed creaking. Not a single hint until months later, after the burial, when a loca cleaning the room found a dried condom with Sergio's snot, and took it to be buried in la Regine's tomb.

HOT PANTS AT THE SODOMY DISCO

On the edge of the Alameda, practically bumping up against the old Church of Saint Francis, the gay club flashes a fuchsia neon sign that sparks the sinful festivities. An invitation to go down the steps and enter the colorful furnace of music-fever sweating on the dance floor. Where the fairy parade descends the uneven staircase like goddesses of a Mapuche Olympus. High and mighty, their stride gliding right over the threadbare carpet. Magnificent and exacting as they adjust the safety pins in their freshly ironed pants. Practically queens, if not for the loose red stitches of a quickie fix. Practically stars, except for the fake jeans logo tattooed on one of the asscheeks.

Some are practically teenagers, in bright sport clothes and Adidas sneakers, wrapped in springtime's pastel colors, healthy glow on loan from a blush compact. Practically girls, if not for the creased faces and the frightful bags under their eyes. Giddy from rushing to get there, they show up tittering each night at the dance cathedral inside the basement of an old Santiago cinema, where you can still see the black and gold Etruscan friezes and Hellenic columns, where the stench of sweaty seat cushions hits hard once you finally get past the burly bouncer at the door. That's where spongers circle, hovering around any gay man who might cough up their cover. We'll figure it out inside, they croon into ears with little dangly earrings. But the gays know that, once inside, the most they'll get is ". . . have we met?" because every taxi boy heads straight to the bar, where the grannies flaunt their piggy banks, rattling ice in a glass of imported whisky.

The bar at a gay club is a good place to meet someone, the area with the best light for spotting the witch who never sees the sun, always underground like the roots of an AIDS-ridden philodendron. The same one who cried sapphire tears, forgiving herself for all her dirty tricks, the spitting in drinks, the broken condoms, the falsified positive test results that aided and abetted a few girls' suicides. Her schemes for infecting half of Santiago because she didn't want to die alone. It's that I have so many friends, she said. The same Miss Perverse who's back again, more alive than ever, laughing luciferously with a drink in hand.

Here's where they pour the gin and tonics, pisco sours, pisco sores, pisco-colas and loca-colas singing along to "Desesperada" by our darling Marta Sánchez, which always makes the disco babes go crazy. The girls in shorts who come up to the bar breathlessly asking for water with ice, elbowing the office worker who's still wearing his tie and who keeps eyeing the door in case someone from his work shows up.

The club bar is for trading glances and putting one's erotic goods on display in certain preferred brands of clothing—the ones that can be found at a thrift store, anyway. A Levi's patch guarantees a luxury booty—a pair of cowboy glutes bursting out of its seams, fibrous in the tight motion of resting both cheeks against the bar counter. Practically masculine, if not for all the ironing and that soft detergent smell. If not for the hand-stitching inside the seams. Way too clean, like trying to make up for something, justifying their homosexuality in the powder-puff aroma that frames their movements. If not for those dense clouds of pansy perfume: Addiction by Paloma Picasso, Obsession for Men by Calvin Klein, Orpheus Rose by Paco Colibrí. If not for those aromatic names emanating from their aerobic stupor, they'd pass as extremely friendly heterosexual men, for sloshed little machos drooling on their buddies. If not for that "Ay, honey, I warned you," "Ay, Chela, you deserved it, you witch," "Ay, if only," "Ay, don't you think?" If not for the "Ay" that crowns or decapitates every sentence, they'd blend right in with the hordes at any old discotheque, dressed in denim and a white shirt with that little crocodile gnawing at the nipple.

Though gay discos have existed in Chile since the seventies, and only in the eighties institutionalized as a backdrop for the gay cause, mass-producing the Travolta model for men and men only. It's possible that these homo-temples of dance have united the gay ghetto with far more success than militant politics, imposing certain lifestyles and a philosophy of macho camouflage that uses fashion to dress the full spectrum of local homosexualities in a single uniform. The folkloric fairies and freaks have survived only as little baubles hanging on homo culture, under the delusion of being a pharaohess fluttering in the dance club's mirrors. A last dance that squeezes last sighs from a loca overshadowed by AIDS. The hot coal of a loca show that the gay market consumes in its business of sweaty muscles. Potentially only that spark, that humor, that argot makes for a politicizable distance. A wildflower petal drifting forgotten on the dance floor when the sunrise cuts off the music and their laughter, in a pale return to the city's routines, blurs with the traffic on the Alameda.

FALSE LASHES

Funerals for sick locas have transformed into a social event. A runway show of exquisitely selected, newly debuted Calvin AIDS models, all giving their friend what she deserves, a send-off like she never dreamed of in Neverland's golden airport.

That plague stigma, which in the eighties made friends flee like rats, denying a thousand times they'd ever known the victim. That virulent homophobia, which back then meant three or four people poor enough to skin cats walking behind a plain coffin. A sad box with tolerant family members standing around, plus some anonymous loca camouflaged in a suit and sunglasses. But everyone's a real social butterfly these days. In the nineties, it's an event the whole audience looks forward to, all waiting patiently for the sick girl's demise in order to wear a little number saved especially for a tragic premiere.

Now AIDS burials fall into a hierarchy. Not just anyone can bid the world goodbye with the Hollywood glamour that carried off Hudson, Perkins, Nureyev, and Fassbinder. Not just anyone can pull off that leopard-spots look, a spreading tattoo that doesn't fade, mind you. That's why the momentary brilliance of the AIDS adiós is unforgettable. It's a rendezvous of broken eyelashes and smothered tutu giggles. It's the moment we've all been waiting for—paying tribute to the deceased as she shows off that pallid, neo-Gothic face of hers. Her huge violet bags match the discreet handkerchief that will dry a single tear in a single moment of throwing a single rose—no, a single petal—on the polished coffin.

This is how the locas, draped in drama, have made a flamenco tablao out of their death, a catwalk mocking sordid funeral rites. Or rather, that in refusing the compassion that weighs like condemnation on the homosexual disease, they transform it into allegory. With all the swish of switchgrass, they cushion the pain, coloring it, polishing it, releasing it from that pious stink. They let it shine in the comic opera of their wail. And no one knows if the diamond tear that rolls down her cheek is authentic. Who could question that bitter theatrical teardrop, which shines like a sequin in the final scene. Those slightly trembling hands, which measure every sigh, every condolence, as if tailoring an evening gown. As if each gesture of pain were being quilted into pleats of sorrow, stitches of forbearance, adjusted and held up by pins of pansy collusion.

A loca dead from AIDS lives only for the camera. Her fidgeting friends attend the event, trying to tie their braids with nervously solemn ribbons. Distracted, they watch the clock, thinking that the list keeps getting longer. "One good turn deserves another" is the funeral oration. No one knows who has a ticket booked on Gotcha Airlines, Boeing Seven-Sero-Positive. No one can laugh all that much. Especially not that scrap of a girl with hair like an angel, who made a show of fainting in the cemetery, keening like an asthmatic dog, it was enough to break your heart. Especially not her, who, right before they shut the coffin, as if by accident, knocked some cigarettes and matches inside, since her friend never did sleep well without a smoke.

LOBA LAMAR'S LAST KISS
("SILK RIBBONS AT MY FUNERAL, PLEASE . . .")

She had street smarts and a genius for her own behind in flaunting that name, that triumph of maritime vaudeville that crowned the dance floor the moment it left the announcer's lips. The brasses blaring out "Mambo No. 8," the bloody wink of the spotlights, the hands clapping her onstage. Those hands slapping her skinny man's ass as it shook to the beat of the tambourine.

She went by Loba Lamar, the Sea Lioness, maybe for the wet grime of her dark skin, for the olive algae of her pelt that the sailors wrung out every night. But Loba Lamar was more than that: a teardrop of black lamé, the trampled embers of a travesti Africa, a dark glimmer among the harbor lights. She used to trip on the stairs as she retraced her path up the hill to her seedy rented room, tumbling onto the steps amid peals of drunken laughter and the sharp smell of belladonna. It was hard to keep upright at that hour, after having mamboed through the night in those unmistakable stilettos. After weathering the seasickness of AIDS, clouding it over by mistaking the sea for the sky, which splashed a vertigo of stars against the waves. In those moments, Loba believed that it had all finished oh so quickly, oh so painlessly, oh so suddenly, that an AIDS death was just a missed step on the dance floor, a path of sparks over the Caribbean like a passage to another world. A moon in the water, caught in tropical currents, beyond the epidemic's reach. But morning always found her there just the same, leaping from star to star. Her missed step was not death, more like a pale return to her destitute life as an unsung loca.

Lobita never understood what being a carrier meant, which was lucky, or AIDS would have taken her straight down on its depressive toboggan. But Loba didn't have much of a head for connecting her own positive result with the drama of disease. She thought everything was fine, there was no convincing her that this check mark was an eviction notice. And though she turned and turned the report card between her fingers, the arithmetic of converting plus to minus didn't enter her head, and her little bird brain never solved the math problem, never drew those little boxes that help you add and subtract. Loba was always a hopeless loca, rubbish at her studies and bullied at school. A plus could no less subtract than a minus could ever add up, and up yours with those numbers and to hell with life. And if I won a prize, she said, this paper isn't going to convince me.

We never saw Loba sad, but a dark cloud bloomed in her yerba maté that day. She folded the sheet and took a deep breath, inhaling the room's stale air. She gulped and sighed until the stench overwhelmed the gravity of the news. Then she walked to the window and opened it, looking out over the rusting seaside roofs. She took a lock of her hair, faded by cheap dye, and yanked it out, making a sound like ripping paper. She watched it flash copper in a ray of sunlight reflected by the glass. Then she opened her hand, letting the strands float into the feathered breeze that cushioned the afternoon.

La Lobita never let emaciation ruin her looks. As she yellowed, she added rouge; the bigger her bags, the bigger her smoky eyes. She never let herself go, not even in those final months, when she was a string of a body, her cheeks stuck to the bone, her scalp shining through a downy fuzz of hair. Even then she looked bronzed by the sun, "though my heart is in winter," a line she tirelessly repeated in her variety show, when fatigue no longer let her dance.

For us, the locas who shared her room, Loba had made a

pact with the devil. How has she lasted so long? How does she still look pretty with those scabs falling off like petals? How, how, how? No AZT, just spunk and her own pulsing heart, and boy did her stubborn ass resist. It was the sun, the good weather, the heat. She withstood the whole summer like a cherry, the whole fall which was warm, and only as winter arrived, as the harbor rain began to drizzle its numbing brine, only then did she show symptoms of goodbye. She fell onto her cot and never got up again. And so the agonies began.

Lobita never wanted to go back to the doctor after that first exam. He's in bed with the gravedigger, she said. She couldn't stand those health centers either, which she thought looked like leper concentration camps. Like in *Ben-Hur*, the only movie she'd ever seen in her entire life. She remembered perfectly that part when Charlie Heston goes looking for his mother and sister in the leper colony. And they both hide, not wanting the boy to see them like that, stripped of skin, their flesh falling off in chunks. Because they had been so beautiful, gorgeous, real nice-looking, though never nearly as nice as Loba, who spent whole nights delirious, recounting the movie. Burning with fever, she cursed the Roman galleys together with Ben-Hur. And she made everyone who was perched on her cot row along with her, threatening to drown herself as the hot waves of her temperature made her shout, Attention, whores of the oar! Onward, maracas of mambo!

We took shifts caring for her, washing her bum like a baby. We were her nannies, her nurses, her cooks, a troop of slaves she bossed around with her Cleopatra airs. We were so patient with her, we would count to twenty, twenty breaths to stop ourselves from wringing her neck. If she'd only shut up and let us sleep a little. At least an hour, during all those insomniac nights on her deathbed. Her demented condition of moribund queen, refusing to kick the bucket and wanting every little thing, every eccentric whim satisfied. One midnight, in the rainy depths of winter, she wanted fresh peaches. And like idiots we left the house in the downpour, all of us wetter than pelicans, rummaging for change as we searched the deserted streets, waking up every shopkeeper in the port, going up and down the hills until we found a can of the damned fruit. And when we returned, shaking ourselves dry like dogs, la Loba chucked the can at our heads because her craving had come and gone. Now she wanted tangerine ice cream. Tangerine ice cream? Can't you want something else, honey? They don't make tangerine ice cream in Chile, Lobita, understand. But she insisted that it had to be tangerine, threatening to die right then and there if she couldn't smell that spring fruit's bittersweet perfume. And in the middle of June, frostbitten with cold, the locas turned around and went out again, braving the elements until they found a slick-eyed Argentine who, after hearing them wail the dying mamacita tango, agreed to sell them a cone. But even then Lobita couldn't sleep, now fixated on the pink flesh of a summertime melon. Ay! sighed the faggot over the sweetness of a cantaloupe, as if she feared not living to see January. As if she couldn't leave this world with that craving still drying her mouth. Because in hell there are no peaches, or tangerines, or melons. And that much heat makes you thirsty.

Ay! Slaves of Egypt, bring me melons, grapes, and papayas, raved the poor thing, waking the whole boardinghouse with the cries of her queenly pregnancy. As if the disease's holocaust had become a gestation of grief, swapping life for death, birth pangs for the throes of agony. The deranged Loba transformed AIDS into a promise of life, imagining that what she carried was a child incubated in her anus by her lost love's fatal semen. That prince of Judea, Ben-Hur, who had planted the fruit in the Roman galleys one night and then left at dawn, leaving her pregnant in a sinking ship.

Night after night we heard her call him, as we tried to placate Loba's parturient cravings. Because then she insisted we make clothes and a cradle for this prince she was bringing into the world. She set us all to knitting little sweaters and hats and vests and booties for her baby. She made us sing lullabies, rocking her as we fanned her with feathers, as if we truly were the slaves of an expectant Nefertiti. At some moment or another she had managed to cast us in her movie, so convincingly acted that, drained by exhaustion, we, too, came to believe in the coming delivery. So all the locas kept getting up in the freezing cold, sneezing, listening to her psych-ward fantasies, her final dalliances, her little voice strangled by coughing fits, more muffled each day but still shrieking orders. Until one afternoon, still haughty, she opened her mouth like a hippopotamus on the Nile and no sound came out. She was struck dumb in her pharaonic command. And there we sat, waiting, covering the mirrors so that Loba wouldn't look at herself again. Begging, praying, pleading for that airplane from nowhere to arrive soon. Mopping her sweat, saying Ave Marias and reciting rosaries like background music. All of us there, paler and shakier than Lobita herself, awaiting the minute, the second, in which this loca would sigh her last breath and our prayers could cease. The whole holy night spent watching her face, which to tell the truth looked more gorgeous than ever. Her silk skin, like a black tiger lily, rippled with light in that abyss. Her swan neck of dark pearl drooped like a ribbon. Then a cold breeze blew through the window, as if someone had opened a tomb. La Loba tried to say something, call someone, modulate a scream out of those tensed lips. She opened her rolling eyes, trying to snatch one last photo postcard from life. We watched how she flapped, desperate not to be swallowed by the shadow. We felt an icy touch that left us stiff, unable to do anything, unable to look away from Lobita, her jaw wide open but unable to let out a scream. We stood there like idiots, shocked by the dark corridor of her mouth, open like a black hole, like a cesspit in which we could just glimpse her prattling tongue. Her bottomless mouth paralyzed in the immense "AH" of a silent opera. Her marvelous mouth unchained like the entrance to a tunnel, like a sewer drain that had carried Lobita into the foul waters of that whirling, sinister eddy. And only then did we react, only then did we run to the edge of that ditch, shouting down, Don't die, Lobita darling. Don't leave us, beautiful. Sobbing, still horrified by her mouth, we stuck our hands into that darkness, trying to grab her by the hair as she fell. All of us struggling to reach her, to drag her back into the living. We grabbed her hands, rubbed her feet, shook her, embraced her, covered her in kisses, sissies crying in unison, sissies laughing neurotically, sissies bringing her water, pushing her, not knowing what to do or what to serve our guest, Señora Death, who was calling at such a disagreeable hour.

And we saw our friend depart on that river of weeping, on that trusty diseased glider carrying her open-mouthed to heaven. She can't go like that, the poor thing, said the locas, already calmer. She can't get stuck with her trap open like a hungry frog, herself so divine, so careful with every gesture and pose. She should always be remembered as a diva. Something must be done. Quick, close her mouth with a scarf before it stiffens. One long enough to wrap around her chin and knot on top of her head. Not yellow, stupid, what a depressing color. Not polka dots either, she'd look like a cartoon, and Lobita would never have worn that. Green? Worse, she hated the cops. Sky blue? Nuh-uh, she's no premature baby. What about that turquoise chiffon with gold thread, yes that same one you're hiding you faggot piece of shit with your friend here dead. This looks fabulous on her yes and wraps all the way around her jaw and there's even enough for a bow. Don't knot it on her forehead, for the love of God, the ends look like rabbit ears and turn her into Bugs Bunny, the poor dear. And don't put the knot under her chin either, as if she were Heidi or some Russian babushka. Better on the side, near her ear, like how Lola Flores wore it, back when they called her the Pharaohess, Lobita thought the world of her. A nice, tight knot, even if it crushes her cheek, leave her jaw shut for an hour at least, until it sets and hardens. So for an hour the locas busied themselves bathing the corpse in enough milk and starch for a Babylonian queen. They smeared her with boiling wax, leaving her hairless and slicker than a nun's tit, while someone else gave her a manicure, gluing on little mollusk shells like fake nails, and another sawed off her calluses and bunions, scaling off the calcified grime of her feet. Because you, dearie, were like Christ, who walked across the sea without touching water. Gordita, you were never all that black, you just roly-polied in the dirt, too lazy to wash with soap, always applying rouge and perfume over the muck, said the locas, scrubbing Lobita with chlorine. While they were waxing her eyebrows and curling her lashes with a heated spoon, the dead queen began to go stiff. So they untied the knot mooring her face to do her makeup and discovered with glee that the scarf had closed her mouth as tight as a crypt. But just when the locas touched her cheek, Loba's lips opened into the macabre smile of rigor mortis. Ay no, shouted one of the queens, she can't go looking like that, with a vampire grin. Something must be done! Bring hot towels to soften her up. Make them practically boiling, the girl can't feel a damn thing. But the heat from the rags made a nerve spasm and her jaw dropped again, her lips opening into a cackle. Looks like our girl is having a laugh at our expense, growled la Tora, the Bull, a burly loca who'd been a wrestler when she was younger. Leave her to me. And we kept quiet because an angry Tora is a serious thing. We meekly reminded her to do it with love. Remember, she's quite frail, amiga. Don't worry, said la Tora, snorting, she's not going to beat *me*. We watched her disappear before coming back sheathed in her lucha libre attire, with her scarlet cape and devil mask that had earned her the nickname Lucifer, The Un-fallen Angel, The Invincible Flame. After warming up with a few jumps and a couple of shark attacks, la Tora asked us to clap for her. And in the midst of that Andalusian bullring hullabaloo, her face turned suddenly serious and she cut off the cheers with a shh of silence so she could concentrate. Not even a fly buzzed as she knelt at the foot of the bed and ritually crossed herself, as she would before entering the ring. And with a leap she was on the cadaver, pummeling it with knuckle-bruisers. *Paf, paf,* the sound of punches filled the room until Loba's face looked like mashed potatoes. Then la Tora lifted her hammy fist and, with her thumb and index finger, squeezed Lobita's cheeks together hard until her lips whistled into a rose. Suck your molars, dearie, suck your molars like Marilyn Monroe, la Tora said, not moving her hand. She kept those cheeks pressed between her pincers for almost an hour, waiting until Loba's flesh returned to its mournful rigidity. Only then did she let go, and we could see the marvelous result of her necrophiliac handiwork. There we stood, hearts in our hands, all of us teary-eyed as we gazed at la Loba, who threw us a kiss with her puckered smacker. We should cover up the bruises, someone said, reaching for her Angel Face powder. But why bother, when pink and lilac go so well together?

POST-90

FROU-FROU EXILES
(THERE WAS ONCE A CAFÉ IN MONTPARNASSE)

Maybe the exiles who returned to Chile right as democracy rose once again over the cordillera brought a new social class back with them, a class that over the years had spread their sorry tale across the world, orphans beaten and cast out from their homeland who found asylum beneath foreign solidarity's sensitive wings. Maybe the Chilean exiles who left the country one bitter morning with nothing but the clothes on their backs nevertheless possessed, at that time, certain political or cultural privileges, free to choose the embassy and the destination that matched the European landscape shimmering in their dreams. Unlike everyone else, the anonymous downtrodden who landed wherever they were thrown: Mexico, Argentina, Cuba, or faraway Scandinavia, where they were just charcoal roaches in the Vikings' albino sky.

But for those who had friends and family in "cultural" Europe, it wasn't hard to make do as intellectual exiles who toured museums in Florence and studied at the Sorbonne, turning into Frenchies who spoke that gargle of a language while fanning themselves with a Chilean newspaper on some boulevard, sighing over the black days that we, their compatriots, were suffering in Chile, in military shit up to our necks and bullets wiping our asses.

Many of the elite's exiles became artists or writers in those evening salons of patriotic nostalgia. Many believed that distance and inspiration were synonyms, stimulated by rosé and Benedetti poems. And when the nightmare ended, some of them came back with certain international airs—with a certain pride in knowing the world, talking among themselves, remembering those amazing pastas that the Inti would whip up in dear old Italy, or Charo's frou-frou ribs in Paris. They returned with inflated heads, wearing three-piece white linen suits and smoking out of a pipe, invading the resistance's artistic scene, which according to them was a cultural blackout where nothing had ever happened.

For those of us who'd wept along with the chords of "Cuando me acuerdo de mi país," we never imagined the exiles would return transformed into a political class that trotted out colonizing habits picked up in the Old World—perhaps yes, a little to adapt, but then quite a bit more for having been cultural climbers from the start.

For this generation that watched the smoke from the protests on satellite TV, coming back was a cinematic *THE END* for their arthouse film, a farewell on a bridge over the Seine, the dregs of a tango drunk with goodbyes on the Champs-Élysées. An ominous return flight to the poor Pudahuel airport, which, no matter how much they improve it, continues to be a ridiculous mall plopped in the dust-winds on the city outskirts. Almost a telephone booth, a toy airport compared to Oslo, Zurich, or Fiumicino. It almost makes me want to turn around when I see the real Chile, so poor and ugly. Nothing like the land my parents yearned for back in Copenhagen. And I say: What the hell did they think they were going to find in this pigsty to begin with?

So exile was not just a forced separation from habits and landscapes; for many of the young people born on European sheets, upon confronting their humble provenance, it also sparked a certain kind of rejection. Because though they might have peasant faces with stiff manes of hair, they find it hard to think of themselves as Chilean, having spent half their lives cradled in the Old World's guarantees. Something of that stateless sophistication is understandable in the children, but not in their parents, who brought even their French soup recipes back with them so they could sprinkle their soirées with chives and the music of Bécaud, Prévert, and Piaf. When the Wall fell and the Left's utopias wobbled and lurched, these home-again snobs were surely the first people to swap their red overalls for a modern miniskirt. The first to adopt the cultural bourgeoisie's prettified politics, with their little rites and rituals. Just like those aristocrats educated in Europe a hundred years ago, the Red-Lights make every gathering unbearable, talking only to each other, reminiscing in whiny French, Do you remember, Katy, that café in Montparnasse? Oh Maca, I remember that night with Silvio, los Quila, and la Isabel. It was the best. So all the Do you remembers, I remembers, How could I forgets frivolize the Chilean exile's bastard movie into bubbles of champagne. They taint with tourism the involuntary uprooting of so many others who were desperately homesick, dying to return and sunk by the abysmal impotence they felt as the curtain of grief fell over their eyes. So many others, famous or not, doubly exiled by suicide, terminal illness, or the bottomless depression of asking each day: Did you get a letter? I know. Yes, they told me already. Exile's other half, who lived out their expulsion organizing peñas, kneading empanadas until dawn, or collecting funds to support the homeland combatants' resistance—they are the silent returnees who rarely invoke the expat melancholy of wandering far and wide, who never got used to it, the insomnia night after night of waiting for reentry paperwork, who came back without making a fuss and had to learn to live with that incurable crack in their hearts.

These days the Left's golden boys are a chummy group of exile's alumni, who strut their social and economic achievements at tacky political events. Perhaps they always wanted to belong to this world of jet-setters who flash their teeth in fashion magazines. Maybe they'd always looked with secret admiration at the bourgeoisie's feather boas, which communist ideology deprived them of. In short, this past century's final decade has spoiled the whiskquierda's ethical trump card, as it watches the millennium's death throes with ice in its heart and a marron glacé stuffed up its nose to ward off the past's mortuary stink.

THE BALLAD OF WILLY ODDÓ

(OR, A TRAVESTI MAIDEN'S MORTAL SCRATCH)

And worst of all it was rush hour when the funeral cortege proceeded through the downtown streets, the purple dye still drying on their flags. Like a parenthesis in history, they picked their way between street vendors, honking buses, and the strangled cries of the Communist Youth, who didn't stop singing "The Internationale" at the top of their lungs. No rhyme or reason, no sense of where to put the emotion, on which phrase, on which rallying verse of that glorious march. Lost and uncertain, they didn't know where to place the accent of their rage, where to mention who murdered Willy, dead at the hands of the pimped and travesti night.

The outpouring was not nearly as huge as for leftist funerals during the old dictatorship. Barely half a block of famous faces flat from the shock. A couple of politicians, some actor on TV, and street theater's boisterous troupe of masks, stilts, and acrobats. All of them had known Willy Oddó, a lead singer of Quilapayún, the pioneering band that played revolutionary Nueva Canción music, Willy, who had only just returned to a democratic Chile, only just settled back in Santiago, where he was still trying to square this shitty modern city with the shtetl he'd left behind as a political refugee, where he now had so many plans and projects as the municipality's new cultural attaché. And so he'd spent his days driving around in his little car, talking to everybody, gathering a record of what had happened in the country while he'd been away. Because truth be told, this was a Chile that Willy didn't know at all, not after so many years abroad singing the same songs, the same "Plegaria a un labrador" for gringos in solidarity. The same chant of *el pueblo unido jamás será vencido*, which so thrilled the Italians sucking up their saucy spaghetti. Little Luchín's same muddy bum for the chic and elegant French. The same banshee yips and wails of Violeta Parra, rehashed a thousand times for European piety. The same planes, the same stadiums and concerts full of exiles singing the woe-is-me cueca, eating artificial empanadas and humitas made from frozen corn. He'd circled the world like that, like the red dove cast out from the ark who never came across its island. And later, after the Flood, having just returned from decades of singing the Chilean martyr's protest songs, what is he confronted by but this tango death, a street fight ripped straight from the pink pages. A death with no ideology, from another kind of musical score, a bolero of alcohol and witching-hour euphoria. Because Willy never dreamed that one Saturday night the city would be carrying a knife between its breasts.

Willy would never again be as happy as he was at that last party. It was the last time he would be so good-looking, with the silver foxiness of a poet who sets great feats to music. With so many friends, so much running into each other again, so many weird artists and cultural figures who drank and drank, clinking glasses for post-90 Santiago. After the liquor ran out and everyone left for some hip basement to keep partying, our Willy needed to extend his embrace even further, into the city's lustful and unshodden streets. He still hadn't spoken face-to-face with her when she was pricked by night's roving desires.

Flooring the accelerator, he zoomed toward Plaza Italia, the epicenter of all the marches, the diva of secret meetings, the star of NO, where the plebiscite campaign hoisted its first flag. Where the packed bar Prosit still emitted fumes of beer and sodomite faggotry. And there, just below the bright blue neon sign, was a cruising ladybugger selling her seventeen summers of travesti charm. So young that from a distance she passed for a woman. So sleek and hairless that, in the dim light, even dressed like a man she passed for a miss, the saucy minx, so girlish and young but already prancing about.

And maybe if her fairy heels hadn't struck sparks on that pavement, summoning him, maybe if Willy hadn't seen her, slamming the brakes to throw her in. Like in that song by Serrat about kidnapping a mannequin, or like bringing a late-night crowd to its knees with a Luis Miguel cover. And if it had been just that, a line from a song, a metaphor that slips past, a pearly desire on a face that fades into traffic. If the light hadn't been red—on top of everything it was red. Perhaps if the punk had known who Willy was, if at some point she'd happened to hear Quilapayún in the reverberations of her club culture. Or if at least they hadn't chilled the romance of it all by discussing her rates. If they hadn't broached the price of flesh, with *todos los pobres del mundo* as the soundtrack. That tension of so much for how much, the tussle, the haggling, the look you pay me or I get out. Because the runny-nosed thing didn't have any romantic notions that could throw her prostitute dealings off course. She had a family to take care of, and that's why she was out working. She didn't have time to talk of yesterdays, and even less to listen to protest songs, and she told him so:

And he seemed not to hear her
And she gulped, she was sullen
And he gazed out the window like nothing
And she insisted about the money
And he laughed, thinking it wasn't about that
And she wanted to get out of the car
And he grabbed her by the shoulder
And she reached for something in her purse
And he'd only wanted to embrace her
And she hadn't understood
And he stretched out his arm
And she plunged the knife beneath the arm of Willy Oddó.

Because she never meant to kill him, she said, the little punk, trembling on TV. Only to cut him somewhere so he'd get scared. Which is why she fled, not knowing her humble pocketknife had sliced an artery that drains the body of blood in five minutes. *La vida no era eterna*, just like that Víctor Jara song says. Because bad blood in the land of milk and honey flows just the same. She with her few short years already knew that. That's why when she faced the press she came clean. Or rather, her deadly adolescence had trapped her, she was a prisoner of the whorehouse night and its bleak future. She sang her life's story as if dubbing a song. She told them every detail, omitting nothing, and bore on her illiterate shoulders the responsibility of having murdered a legend. She faced the electric jolt of flashing cameras, docile, submissive, and nervous as she posed. She ran, almost naively, the gauntlet of the Left's hate as if parading beneath a pink barrage of copihue flowers. By saying no, she said yes. But she insisted that it wasn't a political crime.

And for such a fine televised performance, they gave her many years in prison. Extra vacation in the penitentiary, on that grim patio where all the loca convicts hang out. She didn't have any trouble there, running into old girlfriends on their rusty skates behind the iron bars. Nor was it tricky, being so young, to find herself a beau in that jungle of machos tamed by confinement. And easy as anything, as if having stepped on a piece of gum, the shadow stuck to her, and grew and spread there like mold on the walls. When it rains it pours, the schoolgirl travesti had learned as a little girl. So those terminal catacombs didn't seem quite so terrible to her—not the shrieks in the middle of the night, or the brushstrokes of blood that decorated the cells.

Maybe after she heard Quilapayún on the cassettes the political prisoners had lent her. After listening to hours of *En esa carta me dicen que cayó preso mi hermano*. Perhaps she came to know a Willy who, at some other time, she'd have wanted to meet. And it's possible this is why she accepted AIDS like a double sentencing, soulful and private, thinking that life was wise, but also so unfair sometimes, if what goes around comes around only once you've caught the bird in your hand, and slit its throat with the caress of a knife.

AFTERTASTE

Spending the afternoon in Bellavista with the photographer Álvaro Hoppe, after we roamed over the uneven thresholds of its sidewalks warmed in the burnished cast of twilight, after we reminisced, unsentimentally, about the vertigo of the eighties and the dictatorship's final years, when Hoppe, in air thick with tear gas, sweated his eyes out taking photos of the clashes in the street. Just as I ask him, with democratic ease: Do you miss those days and all that hairy rumbling? And Álvaro can barely reply, drowned out by the vibrating thrum of a helicopter that roars above us and heads straight for the Pío Nono Bridge, where a strangely agitated crowd is stirring behind the railings, running, crossing intersections against the red light, shoving each other right up to the edge of the Mapocho River swamped with police and wailing patrol cars with their lights also flashing red. So many pairs of eyes watching the water, shouting: Over there! Over where there's a shoe floating, a foot, a leg, a hand, and then a head that surfaces in the muddy current before sinking again into the mouth of dark chocolate. It's a man. It's a boy. No, it's a woman, say the onlookers when the firemen and police pull her limp body out and up to the bridge, where an improvised emergency team tries to wrench her back from death, giving her mouth-to-mouth, pumping her chest to force water out of her lungs, raising and lowering her arms, which only flop back to the cement. Over there's another one! Over there a body bobs up for a moment, like a marionette swaying in the water, then sweeps under the bridge, submerged, and we all move to a different railing in time to see the wobble of a baby shoe sucked down by the spiraling current. On the other side of the street, the woman has died, and policewomen dressed like men cordon off the scene with yellow tape, which frames the cadaver now covered in funereal plastic. A cruel, lively spirit runs through the onlookers crowded on the bridge, whispering: This looks like '73. First to find a body wins a prize. It's overflow from the twin towers. Downstream, firemen grab for the swift unraveling bundles that are soon lost to the Mapocho's frothing, frilly shroud. And that's when I remember I have an important errand to run, and I say goodbye to Álvaro, who stays a minute longer, captivated by what's unfolding.

That night I get home and turn on the TV, but what we saw evidently wasn't worth making a fuss over, swallowed by the latest reports from Afghanistan and the capture of a psychopath who murdered seven girls up north. The news anchor, her voice laden with professionalized concern, says that a woman by the name of Nadia Retamal Fernández threw herself into the Mapocho today, along with her two small children, Daniela and Brian. All three drowned to death. We'll be back after this commercial break. Then a nausea of possibilities blurs the screen as I can't unhear what sounded like a moral condemnation of this woman's decision to commit suicide, of the deflated corpse I saw that afternoon and whose name I now know: Nadia Retamal Fernández, maybe young, perhaps dragging a sack of grief that allowed no second guesses when she jumped. And it's possible that in her final seconds she wished for a gust of luck from the future to hold her back. A warm wind that she dreamed could close the hungry mouths of her children, Daniela and Brian. Perhaps on that sharp edge of the abyss she didn't want to hear the president's speeches echoed back at her, talking about economic miracles and the breadcrumbs our nation hands out to the poor. Maybe at this last stop she held her kids tight and the only piece of them she kept was the wild fluttering of their little hearts. And, in judging her for the infanticide, there's a good chance we will fail to understand what motivated her, or even begin to appreciate her desperation—which, like a flag on a sinking ship, slips into the depths of the coastal afternoon just moments before the glare off our great homeland blocks out the sun.

GONZALO
(MEMORY'S COMPACT)

As if no one could remember his elephantine silhouette powdering the dictatorship's face, covering that crack, this crease, that filth in the corner of his mouth, as the tyrant sarcastically wondered on television about the exact number of disappeared. In the depths of emergency blackouts and official decrees, Gonzalo's plump hand lengthened shadows, dusting repression's face with light and coloring it with hypocrisy. Because Gonzalo, effeminate stylist and perpetual admirer of men in uniform, held carte blanche as hairdresser, tailor, and makeup artist to those on high, receiving special clearance to come and go from the commander-in-chief's house. And pity the jarhead who threw him a kiss or made fun of his silk scarves wafting in the powder's smoky haze. Pity the buzzcut who imitated his walk, the way his hips quivered like jelly, their fascist sway that mistook a military parade for a runway show. When he'd walk beneath drawn sabers, head high, flapping his cosmetic case as he paid tribute to the nation.

That's how Gonzalo—or Gonza, as the First Lady would call him, anxious before appearing on television for a national address: Don't you think this flesh-colored Chanel suit is too on the nose for a speech about hunger? Don't you think, Gonza, that this rouge is too red? Ay, Gonza, fix my hat, please, to cover my droopy eye. Ay no, Gonza, don't throw so much blue on me, I'll look like that tart Eva Perón. And so the fantooshed stylist came and went with his Princeton watercolor set, painting sunflowers onto official communications, touching up the barbed wire that surrounded the national landscape, choosing yuppie apple shades to accent the regime's prosperity, radiating summertime strawberries during the harsh authoritarian winter, while bare corpses piled up on the periphery.

No one saw it coming that, when democracy finally arrived, this same figure would be polishing the other side of the coin. No one seemed to notice how, with the ease of a whale, he displaced the political waters. Though the huge void his fatness left elicited sorrow in the army's ranks. Those queers are all traitors, said the ex–First Lady, applying her lipstick herself. Furious with her muddle of rouges and concoctions that she vainly tried to mix to repair the loss. He was shameless, I always knew he was, telling me, Señora Lucy come this way, Señora Lucy over here. My, how fabulous you look in that brown hat, because of your poise, your beauté, your elegance, like a queen who was born to wear a hat.

And so no one knew quite how Gonzalo, taking advantage of the country's amnesia and the Concertación's victory celebrations, switched teams or grabbed onto the conga train welcoming democracy. While everyone's eyes were elsewhere, watching the army's privileged aura grow dimmer, he managed to slip past the chaos by adding some pink to the democratic rainbow.

So he turned up again, spilling out of our small TV screens, offering natural remedies and beauty advice for the new era. His distant love for military style had seemingly vanished. In his voice's fragile tenor, he described his personal friendship with the current president, saying that the Right had suggested he run as a candidate for Colina, but that he'd refused their offer, explaining that he'd only ever been a cadet in the Military Academy, and that the star on the Chilean flag had turned red with envy upon seeing his swan step. But this was all long before the coup, when he was so sleek and slender that he served as a flag-bearer and stood at attention a whole week, planted there in the courtyard. Out of love for his country. Afterward, he said several times that he was not a homosexual, leaving things as clear as there's snow in the Andes. Rather, he explained, he was asexual, which is why adapting to all the political changes came so naturally to him.

Gonzalo's metamorphosis is not immune from judgment, even if his cosmetic sponge is what's sprucing up the new government's two-faced speeches. The grimacing mask that broadcasts its own chipper communiqués to the country. The cardboard face without a face that Gonzalo's plastic fingers adorn with nearly the same formula. Even though it's been years and high fashion's pearly chameleon has updated its colors. And so neoliberalism cross-dresses memory's scars, laying a mask of silver and gold across its uniformly painted eyelids, ready for Carnaval.

SO LONG, CHE!
(OR, A THOUSAND WAYS TO SAY GOODBYE TO A MYTH)

Maybe these days only operatic fanfare can bring to life our past millennium's most troubled periods, which marked the climax in history's own movie. For anyone who lived through the scuffles of the seventies, or read about them in newspapers or books—and for the nineties youth who showed up late and missed the whole revolutionary party—the grand homage to Che in the National Stadium had a sense of resuscitating his memory for a few hours, so that we could finally close the book on such dangerous recollections. For while the event had truly emotional moments, transporting the crowd back to the dictatorship's raw history—and while we must repeat a thousand times the ritual of saying the victims' names and pointing at their executioners—it also must be said that, for the seventy thousand youth who were there, the story of Che was simply one more piece of ancient history invoked to protest the current situation. The air hummed with a deep hatred for the tyrant now entrenched in power, the stands shook with earsplitting condemnations of democracy's neoliberal conditions. That night brought together the whole leftist family with its tireless flutterbutting—the handsome layabouts, the soccer hooligans, the university kids and fiftysomething-year-olds who still listen to Canto Nuevo—as they landed on a way to air their shared disillusionment. And within that framework of rage, grief, and nostalgia, the crowd kneaded each other to the brotherly rocking of *el pueblo unido jamás será vencido*; the masses rubbing up against the chant's political heat, turning the guerrilla's homage into shared ecstasy, a strange mingling of passions in the stadium's cauldron. Not many actually listened to the carefully recited liturgy about Ernesto; even fewer paid attention to the biographical details. And it was better that way, holding on to him as the dreamer of a new world, listening to the letters Che sent his family—documents that now paint him as an old-school macho, telling his wife and daughters to look after the house, to wait for him with dinner hot on the table, and to take good care of his sons, the only ones capable of carrying out the revolution. Surely if Ernesto were alive he wouldn't still be going on about this, wouldn't let them read his personal letters aloud at the ceremony. Maybe he wouldn't even have liked being the star of a mega-event honoring the brief exhumation of his remains. Too many men grasping at the revolution, and quite a few women, too, all reviving that era's macho rhythms. Surely if you were still alive, Ernestito, you'd have taken a harder look at your machine-gun virility. You'd regret that time you threw a book by Virgilio Piñera on the floor in a Cuban embassy library, demanding the ambassador explain what a faggot was doing on the bookshelf. Certainly, if you were alive, you'd be surprised how much your funeral has in common with Princess Di's, and Mother Teresa's, and now, as I'm writing this, with the Spanish infanta's wedding. One big capitalist contradiction. A whole carnival of perplexing funeral rites for the global market. Surely you never imagined it, Ernestito, all those years buried in a secret grave. Surely you never dreamed the world would witness the digging up of your corpse on TV. You'd probably never have agreed to being the guest of honor at this wake for your remains, in a packed stadium, let alone at the funeral in Havana, where even your enemies will purchase box seats. Would you look at that, how the revolution is selling the same spectacle. And I'm not moralizing—just offering another way to look at your legacy, a glance from a sissy sitting among the raving and delirious who chant your name. A glance that's also wet with tears after hearing your voice for the first time when they play a recording over the loudspeakers. Your voice, unfamiliar, but so martial, so militant at a rally way back when, in that distant yesterday, thundering in a speech that I kept hearing even after I left the stadium, after I got lost in a march of seventy thousand souls who that night said goodbye to a myth and opened the door for another Ernesto, more fragile, and warmer, who was knocking shyly at our heart, ready to greet us with a kiss.

DIALOGUE

(OR, DARK NEGOTIATIONS UNDER A WHITE TABLECLOTH)

And it's hard to imagine that Chilean officials would be pushing for this summit between victims and perpetrators, especially the wing of the Concertación that's been trying the hardest to turn the page on the subject of human rights. The families of the detained-disappeared and those responsible for the brutal disappearance sitting before each other, in the same place and with the same guarantees. This creative initiative seems to make the horrific proximity of these crimes even worse by suggesting that the Agrupación de Familiares meet the military lawyers and their foul-smelling fumes face-to-face. Luckily, and with the same dignity that Sola Sierra had maintained for so many years, the association declined to participate in this "table for dialogue," which beneath its democratic tablecloth is hiding a slimy deal.

Pamela Pereira—daughter of a disappeared person and well-known lawyer who has fought for justice for years—was the only one who agreed to share that corrupted and foul air. Salazar did, too, another lawyer who agreed, in a personal capacity, to be a dinner guest at this table of forgiveness, greeting the military delegation and absorbing repression's greasy sweat with each handshake. They're in there, we're out here, those of us who continue to believe that the memory of this atrocity can be met only with justice and with knowing exactly who the slaughterers were.

Maybe the real motivation for the government to reopen the subject is Pinochet's imprisonment in London. Their concerns about getting past these wounds sound an awful lot like a nationalist strategy to liberate the dictator, using this call to brotherhood as part of his defense. Showing the world that Chileans have already dealt with the past's humiliations by bowing our heads. Since we're Christian and civilized, too, and from the third world, and our hearts are such cowardly pieces of shit that we forgive even if they don't ask for forgiveness. That must be why we're able to clink glasses of blood with our executioners on reconciliation's white table. That's why Volodia's son, Claudio Teitelbom, has accepted an invitation to this century's last supper for human rights, a successful young man who appears in the society pages with Andrea Tessa, the musician who sang Pinochet happy birthday. The writer Guillermo Blanco at his side, representing a certain kind of historical fiction that whitewashes everything. And in the center, Pérez Yoma, the government's gloved hand, whose hypocritical sermons all agree we must forget. Farther down there's a priest who sprinkles holy water and, in the name of the bishop, praises gestures of friendships, quiets our resentments, and commands us to turn the other cheek to receive the smack of his benediction. On the other side sit the military's unflappable fuckers, their faces hard with sarcasm and power as they assure us they don't have any specifics about where the disappeared bodies ended up, that no one knows anything, unless this table offers guarantees of absolute protection for any man in uniform who might be willing, as an individual, to share information.

Though they never say it out loud, the word *impunity* pokes out of and twiddles in the generals' ironic mouths. It's more than that—the word *impunity*, though never said out loud, is the only thing that reverberates in this dialogue's conciliatory echoes. Some nervous hand knocks over a glass and stains the ivory tablecloth with big splotches. Another hand with a braided cuff reaches for a canapé and nibbles at its rotting flesh. And outside, in the street, in front of the presidential palace, the blurry faces of the disappeared are pasted on signs that their family members hold against their hearts. And these photos are the only thing left of them, the only thing keeping them here at the edges of this disgusting clique. Maybe in the street, with their faces turned to the sun, illuminating their extinct features, maybe the street is the only place they can be that alive, that direct, like an ethical declaration that exposes the agreement's endgame. They're in there—those who agreed to play a game of poker with marked cards. We're out here, outside the game, with our memories of Sola Sierra, with the mothers and family members and the moral mettle of Viviana Díaz and Mireya García, unshakable in their demand for justice no matter who you are. They're in there, at their long reconciliation table, toasting with wine that impunity has poisoned and breaking the bitter bread of forgetfulness.

ACT LIKE NOTHING HAPPENED, DREAM IT NEVER COULD (AFTER GLORIA CAMIRUAGA'S FILM *LA VENDA*)

She faces the camera head-on, testifying as one among a group of women who survived the cellar of horror. It's less in what she says than in the way she nervously mumbles each word, as she gropes for a way to explain the dark swamp where they were submerged during those days that are so hard to remember yet also seared in some place where memory can draw a blanket over the humiliated sting. This duality, which makes the mind's frayed edges intermittently flinch, seems like the only opening into a certain trembling intimacy of someone shocked even now to be verbalizing these confessions as video testimony. Maybe even just recording these voices makes them louder, women who for many years hid the events in silence, like someone who refuses to recognize the brutal evidence in themselves. Like someone who wishes to never again be caressed by the military glove that stamped her flesh with fingerprint bruises as its patriotic crest. Like someone who finally shows the camera her wounds and their tragic purple emblems, which emerge from the shadows again and again, documenting this country's untold history of torture. The mislaid history of official taunting and government persecution, which has never gone on trial. The corroded history gagged by bureaucracy and democratic indifference.

We need to say a thousand times that this happened, that this took place in neighborhoods not far from here. In front of that plaza where a grandpa now tosses crumbs to the birds. Near the church where a well-groomed priest washes his mouth with the word *reconciliation*. Just beyond the kindergarten, where the same torturer says goodbye to his child with a dirty kiss on the cheek. In that very house, which looks so much like other houses, only with a stench of plague wafting up from the cellar. Family homes right next to these other ones stained with terror, where rust has appeared on sockets that evoke nausea's involuntary shudder. Torn curtains and silent walls where even now you can see scratchings of LAGOS FOR PRESIDENT.

This happened under a heaven that paints its whole hogwash of brothers with the same filthy blue brush. This happened at the foot of a mountain range so white, so proud and pale like a corpse. This happened, and it feels like even by saying so, nothing is said. It appears that in our newly updated atmosphere, these testimonies, inevitably mangled, are now held up as suspect, in need of decoding in a way that whitewashes, muffles, and depoliticizes memory's wet scabs. This happened, these women's moist eyes in the video scream that it happened. This happened . . . but what will it matter if half the country still doesn't believe it? Half the country prefers not to know, not to remember that night when in the house next door, with each electric shock a woman's throat trilled a death rattle of despair. Half the country refuses to believe and wants to turn the page, look to the future, act like nothing happened, dream it never could . . . Half the country doesn't know because they don't want to, they're busy playing dumb. And though it might hurt to say it out loud, the familial complicity of a wife, sister, or mother hiding a son who tortured; the crony ties known as "our fellow countrymen"; the cultural complicity of going wild over art during those black mantle days; the incestuous ruckus on television and the right-wing newspaper goons clinking glasses with the fascist crapola; everything wove a blindfold of individualism that handed monstrous torturers the visa of being a law-abiding citizen.

What the video shows is what can be shown with words, what the naked voices of its protagonists can say. Barely a smudge of bloody residue in the abject hole of their story. The rest of it—what remains, what continues—no sense of solidarity can absorb the total blow of these facts without confronting this country's sham of a democracy in which they are lived out, without feeling again that so many of the people here—out of fear, uncertainty, or indifference—have covered their ears, closed their eyes, and let blindfolds conceal a sky clawed at by the isolated echoes of tortured convulsions.

WELCOME BACK, KING TUT
(OR, THE NIGHTMARE'S RETURN)

This happened quite a few years ago, but the day still feels fresh, that morning when the Air Force's sinister bird crossed into national territory, carrying the decrepit specimen who once represented cruelty and power. As if transporting Tutankhamen's mummy—the aircraft tricked out like a five-star hotel with a lounge, an infirmary, a dining table, and a giant bedroom with a full-size bed, all to carry the grimy dictator like a porcelain doll. And when Augusto Nero felt the aircraft take off from the London airport, when he experienced the sensation of the plane lifting up and hovering in the jet stream, only then did he breathe more easily, thinking that they were taking him to heaven, and he smiled, imagining that there above the clouds he'd find Merino, Leigh, and Mendoza, and that together they'd play a game of dominoes while planning another coup d'état against the eternal Father. As the plane rose into the clouds, Augusto Nero closed his eyes, dreaming that way up there God would personally be waiting for him at the airport gates of Paradise and would decorate him as a saint, naming him commander-in-chief of all the celestial armies. And then he wouldn't have to worry ever again about all those judges and human rights lawyers who persecuted him here on Earth. But when he opened his eyes he knew it couldn't be true, and remembered, bitterly, that he was traveling on a flight back to Chile, where once again a socialist had taken the democratic route and gotten himself elected president. At the thought, he rang the buzzer and called for the nurse, asking her to change the diaper he'd just shat in, to wash his bum and cover it with talcum powder so that he'd arrive in Santiago as fragrant as a newborn babe.

The flight was direct, though the plane made a stop on some tropical islands where Augusto Nero wanted to soak his bunions in the ocean's calypso waters. But no one was there waiting for him, everyone had disappeared from the beaches, scared that old grandpa tyrant would take the island with fire and blood. So the Chilean Air Force flight continued on its way, plowing through the mauve shades of the aurora borealis, while the crew gave Augusto Nero lessons on how to appear extremely ill, making him up to look pale, adding bags under his eyes to foster compassion in the thousands of Chileans who'd woken up at sunrise and turned on the TV, awaiting the return of King Tut.

After landing in Antofagasta, the crew continued en route to Santiago, where the reception's preparations were speeding up, despite the official recommendation that it should be a simple affair. Even so, the military commanders looked like Santa Claus, all buttoned up in uniforms decked with badges and tassels. Behind them, the wives, in their pinochetista Sunday best, their dresses ironed and tailored, eagerly anticipated the return of their stale patriarch. And when the plane touched down at Pudahuel airport, the military band erupted into the "Lili Marleen" march. But the sinister hymn wasn't heard only in Pudahuel; throughout the broadcast, all of Chile—and, thanks to cable TV, the whole world—echoed with the music of the Third Reich. And for a moment the entire planet had a feeling that, in a distant land known as Chile, Hitler was still alive and well, especially when, as the airplane opened its doors, the band launched into "Erika," the Führer's favorite hymn. Luckily it wasn't Adolf who stepped out of the flying machine; in his place was Augusto Nero, the decadent ex-tyrant of Chile, who descended like a virgin on a palanquin, languishing in his wheelchair. And that was when the miracle occurred. Like in his glory days, Emperor Augusto Nero stood up and waddled across the airport runway. The pinochetistas sobbed, the generals' wives applauded ecstatically and looked up at the sky, as if expecting a divine ray of light to shine on the trembling jaunt of the dictator, the same old Augusto Nero who, laughing at the whole world, surveyed his troops, saluted the officers, and, with a final sarcastic smile, climbed into the military helicopter that whisked him off to Hospital Militar, flanked by a thrumming swarm of propellers. Only Rambo and Schwarzenegger were missing when the bulletproof dragonfly landed on the helipad, a battalion of black berets, in combat gear and armed to the teeth, ready to escort him to the building entrance. Gurkhas and snipers stood on the rooftops in the affluent surrounding neighborhood, guarding the place like it was some big-budget cinematic production, a war movie that we were all watching helplessly on our small screens, with a knot in our guts that made us belch with democratic shame.

FINALE

ZANJÓN UPON THE WATER

Dedicated to Olga Marín,
in loving gratitude

ACT ONE:
THE ARCHAEOLOGY OF POVERTY

And who would care if I said that Zanjón upon the Water was where I first saw the light of the world? Who would be interested? Unless they mistake the place for a historical romance novel. But especially if they don't know, will never know, what this arid plot of Chilean poverty really was. Surely without peer among the occupied lands, encampments, and police hot spots in the surroundings of what is now Greater Santiago. But Zanjón—apart from being a legend of population sociology—was also an alley that bordered a horrible canal with the same name. The banks of a swamp where in the late forties they cleared some land, put up pasteboard and tar paper, and overnight there were houses. Shoddy homesteads appeared in every corner like magic, like mushrooms miraculously bursting forth after a storm, blooming between the trash, these precarious shacks were nicknamed toadstools for the way they sprang up in the crannies of all the lackluster bogs in the land.

And of course a place to call home has always been an adventurous excursion for the dispossessed, even more so back then, when entire families from the north and south of the country would immigrate to the capital in search of wider horizons, trying to find a patch of ground where they could plant their borrowed flags. But my family had always lived in Santiago, trading its hide for a room in a boardinghouse or the gray neighborhoods that surrounded the old downtown. Until the afternoon when the eviction came; the cops threw us four mucks into the street, along with the kerosene stove, the wobbly table, the bed frame with its little feet, and a few boxes holding my family inheritance. Maybe someone had told us about Zanjón, and, since we didn't want to sleep outdoors, we went to that sunken beach instead, where the children ran alongside the dogs, chasing rats. And the whole thing was so easy, so quick, that for a few pesos they sold us a wall, not even three square feet of land, it was just a slab of adobe that my grandmother bought. And we built a hodgepodge nest out of that wall, one that sheltered my childhood through each winter and spread its eaves over our tiny family. Starting with that wall—which, like the backdrop of a motion picture, became the facade of our first home—my grandmother added an aluminum roof and a stick frame that held together the flimsy architecture of my childhood palace. But, unlike our neighbors, at least the front of our house sort of looked like a house, at least when seen from the alley, with the window and the door that, opening, revealed a bare floor, there weren't rooms, just an open part at the back where the cold dawn winds came and went like Saint Peter himself.

You'd think that, in recalling those days, I'd feel those shivering childhood mornings as if tattooed on my memory's skin like dry ice. But I was wrapped in maternal harmony's lullaby, safe beneath the umbrella of the proletariat soul. Somewhere in the sawdust clouds and jumble of rotten smells, "I learned the good and knew of the bad." I learned the pride of humble hands, and painted my first tale with the muddy colors and milky sediment that swirled in the Zanjón's waters.

ACT TWO: MY FIRST ECTOPIC PREGNANCY

There's a slogan that goes "Poor, but clean," and maybe it applies in cases where the basics of hygiene are available. But all the water for drinking, cooking, and bathing in Zanjón had to be brought in from an open pit that provided the whole toadstool settlement with its water supply. The wastewater would drain into a foul-smelling gully that ran parallel to the houses, where the women also tossed putrid broth out of piss pots. Stark against that sordid mud, the ivory flutter of sheets and diapers—blindingly white from the boiling bleach—affirmed the scrubbed passion of maternal hands, always bluish, pale, and submerged in soapy wash water. And maybe the only way the Zanjón mothers could symbolically detach from the sludge and the kids dangling in clusters from their sides was through this utopia of whitening, where they latched onto the clouds with the snowy brightness of their dishcloths, the sheets diaphanously unraveling like flags of surrender in survival's own war.

My childhood flitted and fluttered in the sun's swarms of flies, which my mother carefully shooed away until that first distracted moment when, busy with chores, she lost sight of me, and the adventure of crawling out past the toadstools led me to the gully's edge, where I dipped in my little hands, wet my face, and sipped at the sludge in my toddler impulse to learn my environment through taste. And so it was that about a day later my stomach began to swell like I'd been impregnated by the bumblebee prince. More days went by, and the stomach pain and rat-a-tat-tat of constant diarrhea became an unceasing cry. My mother didn't know what to do, rubbing my belly blown up like a balloon and spooning me herbal teas and concoctions of cinnamon and burnt sugar. Back then it wasn't as easy as picking up the phone and calling the family doctor. Especially if you had to get up at five in the morning and leave the house with the wee one clinging to your neck to take a number and wait in the overflowing clinic. But that's how I was delivered into the hands of a doctor with fishbowl lenses, who looked at my poor tummy thinking of African children and their "very typical" malnutrition. But when she pressed on the taut drum of skin, and rested her cold stethoscope against it, a muffled beat startled her, and she drew back, frightened. It's not possible, she told my mother, nervously scribbling a prescription for a noxious purgative. The deliverance happened that night, after I drank the abortive medicine, which stripped my insides in a spasm of diarrhea as florid as marsh water. And there, in the glimmering bedpan's black mirror, floated a tadpole, its minuscule corpse frozen in metamorphosis. Barely more than a head and a tail, though also sticking out were two little green feet, which the baby polliwog had grown inside my gut after I'd swallowed its larva in a microcosm of life that, in spite of everything, was kicking and elbowing its way into a brief window of gestation.

ACT THREE: MEMORIES OF RANCID FLESH

But Zanjón upon the Water wasn't known only for its extreme poverty, for mopping up the sweat and social backwardness of the working class. No, back in the fifties, this fleapit would ink the newspapers with local crimes and a running tally of thugs who took refuge under its corrugated tin roofs. Back then, this pilfering mafia was known as "the shorn," no doubt for the close crop they always got while in jail, their hair shaved off their heads in rough chunks, maybe to make it obvious who they were and that society should reject them. But the shaved-head aesthetic didn't raise eyebrows or cause any discrimination in Zanjón, where it was common to see flea-bitten kids shaved to zero in order to stem the plagues of lice. Besides, it seemed natural that the shorn would come out from behind bars looking like skin-and-bones Jews, bearded and bald, rescued from extermination. A certain familiarity with crime allowed for healthy cohabitation. Because, like any other ecosystem, no matter how tough or slippery you are, there are still laws of brotherhood. It was a kind of moral catechism for them to never ever mug a local resident. Plus, they always lent a hand during the natural disasters that blew the tin roofs off of houses at night. Like how during the floods they bailed out the black water that was pouring into the shacks. And when a huge fire consumed half the neighborhood and no firefighters came, the shorn were our angels of salvation, lugging basins all the way from the well and rescuing babies charred by the flames.

In these social trenches, where huts clung to the miserable edges of the city, a delinquent zoology emerged, each identified according to criminal specialty. The pickpockets, who used their velvet fingers to skim wallets out of purses before shooting off like rockets. The downtown shop girls, like Snooty María, a slippery vampiress who did herself up like a real madam and decimated luxury shops with her double-bottomed purse. The burglar clan, specialists in plundering houses uptown. Sometimes an international shoplifter would pass through on a return trip from Europe, where we exported the Chilean art of the stylish steal. Take Chute the Turd, for example, a svelte dandy who came back smoking Cuban cigars, sporting a white suit and a hat to match. The whole neighborhood welcomed him with a party and a mafioso bender that lasted three days. The little boys were the happiest of all, grabbing fistfuls of coins that Chute threw at them like some stingy godfather. But there were more sinister types, too, like Rancid Flesh, as dark and menacing as a jackal's pupil. He was a wizard at sacking the trucks that drove down Santa Rosa. Rancid Flesh was a single dad, *Kramer vs. Kramer* style, and had dreamed up a trick to stop the drivers who, knowing how dangerous the place was, drove lickety-split through the streets. Whenever he spied a vehicle loaded with goods, Rancid Flesh would throw his seven-year-old onto the highway and the truck would come screeching to a halt, a moment of confusion that let him jump into the back and lighten the truck's load. And maybe there was a time when the driver couldn't stop fast enough and the wheels crushed the runny-nosed kid. But this was an everyday thing in Zanjón, kids dying like stray dogs, being run over in the street. Or killed during police raids, in the middle of the night or at the crack of dawn, bullets that whistled clean through the shacks. The next day the neighbors would rehash the Homicide Brigade's roundup. The Whistler fell last night, they gave it good to Crapjack, Snooty María escaped by a hair, they took Tirifa, Shorty, and Glum-Face away in handcuffs, they shot Jukebox in the foot but he crawled onto the roof, the thieving pigs took a ton of stuff and chalked it up to recovering property. Everyone in Zanjón would be on edge for weeks afterward, sleeping fitfully, afraid the gunshots would return with their indiscriminate fire. And for a while the shorn would vanish into thin air, sometimes immigrating to La Legua or Victoria, where they quietly and carefully continued to perfect the delinquent arts of their trade.

EPILOGUE: NOSTALGIA FOR LOCAL DIGNITY

These days mayors trying to get elected make a big show about new policing methods and lowering crime rates. It's a new era, one where robbery has lost its romance of stealing from the rich to give to the poor, Robin Hood or Jesse James style, maybe because the stars of the social steal are now just runny-nosed kids who grab pensions as the elderly leave the bank. They seem more like thieving rats, lifting bicycles from children and backpacks from students, nothing like those bad boys of yesteryear, Zanjón's subtle vultures who turned life into an adventure novel, transgressing the brutal economic inequality that x-rayed in black and white our country's malnourished landscape.

Now, when poverty dressed in American clothing no longer answers to *pueblo* but hides under the universality of *gente*—more plural, less politicized for filling out those government surveys that distribute welfare to the lowest earners based on the number of appliances in a home. And everything is like that, there are lines of credit for a better life, which let you dream in color as you flip through the catalog, indebted to a well-being paid in installments. To make these times a little easier, to more easily auction off neurons to the television screen, watching the jet-setting fleas fanning themselves with money, having a ball, chewing an olive as they model the latest styles of leisurewear, sticking out their tongues at the terribly crass TV audience who, bleary-eyed, set a casserole dish on the television set to catch the drip leaking from the roof, sounding like coins, which might in their recurring plink be mistaken for the pealing of jewels worn by the crème de la crème, clinking through the screen. But after turning off the TV set, the drip of poverty continues to echo in the empty pot. To more easily survive this era's frosty indifference, fall asleep instead, dreaming the third world was just a broken slipper that washed up on the Zanjón's shores, where a polliwog boy never became a princess who never told the tale of her interrupted croak.

STREET CORNERS OF MY HEART

(OR, NEW KIDS ON THE BLOCK)

This one goes out to the boys in the housing projects, pissing out their drunkenness in the same stairwell where their Beatlemaniac fathers gave it to me doggy-style—shooting myself up, then, with the silvery glint that splashes naked down the steps before pooling in a steaming star. I smoke those vapors with a sigh of love for their rebellious exile. A toast of iodine for their own private world corroded by drugs. In the end, they're so young, disposed by exposure to soaring leaps on the working-class trapeze. A way to kill time wandering with soles stuck on using the same glue that drips deadening into the brain's membranes, opening black holes like windows dressed in mourning or cesspools where you lose yourself until you can barely make out the bulb on the lamppost. Constantly busted, constantly replaced and broken again like trying to nix its status as a halogen recruit, returning the street corner to the old protective darkness of the blackouts, where familiar surroundings transform into a filching wilderness. A mired and swampy anonymity where adolescent faces are traced in fireflies of lit spliffs as they gather under the busted bulb, like turf for lying in wait.

The street corner is a heart where you press your ear, hearing the thumping music that calls people out on a Friday or a Saturday, doesn't matter which; here time marks fatigue in the cracks and badly patched furrows left by the earthquake's shudder. Here time loses the beat in the damp on the walls that haloes faces like candle flames, reflected from window to window, socket to eye socket, surreptitious glances until even the act of looking loses its walled-off autonomy. Here the days drag themselves across staircases and hallways that women mop with hands gashed by bleach as they trade the latest stories about those crazy boys.

The neighborhood corner is the epicenter of lives that barely see the sun, poking their heads out only to cassette the Walkman held together with rubber bands. A pacemaker in your chest so you don't hear the brawls, don't get depressed by the president's bark of laughter when he's asked about young people and their future.

The Walkman is a real cunt of an itinerary, an intercontinental trip bottled along with the pisco so you can pass out with a chorus of Yankee voices promising "this night" or "dis nai." Like this was the last time seeing your old lady's knickers fluttering on the balcony; the last of your neighbor snoring through the plaster wall, the dividing mechanism that the people's architecture came up with as a flimsy support for intimacy, where conjugal gasping and the body's farts and whistles seep from private to public. Like a single reverberation, like a bell clanging neurotically, your mother shouting, your grandpa moaning, the babies crying and sopped in shit. A stuffed bag that pulses with noisy overcrowding where no one can be alone because any person who lives in all that madness opts to jump from the frying pan into the fire of group promiscuity, numbing himself rather than succumbing to squeezing his desires into those tiny rooms. Just a couple yards wide where any shifting means friction, the scuffing of cohabitation. Where any brusque movement rubs a spark that explodes into airing dirty laundry, into how much money is needed before they can hoist the flag for lunch. And the New Kid still sleeping, the lazy bum, hammocked in his drunkenness by Madonna's thighs, which unhook from him right as the shouts begin drilling into his head, right as they throw a "get up, it's noon, for shit's sake" under his door. As if that hour of the day were an instant benchmark for labor's tasks—a bourgeois measure of production for hardworking people who've already earned half a day by then, having gone jogging, walked the dog, and typed out on the computer the whole petty economy of their lives. So that afterward they can complain about a sore back, the prize that the kidneys award to the employee of the month.

How to swap out Madonna's turquoise birthmark for the hairy zits of a middle-aged secretary who sends you wherever she pleases, because you're junior and have to keep your eyes down like you're ashamed. How to swap that old woman's keyboard for the New Kids' mega music, for blacking out deep inside and blowing it all, smoking up to your fingernails and whatever comes, babe, fag, freak, whatever it is, ready to burst with the feeling of it all, you feel me? As long as they don't put on Jim Morrison, because I remember the fucker who froze in the stairwell when it snowed and they found him just like that. A lot of us cried then and some laid down bouquets of marijuana buds, which afterward they smoked right there, saying that anyway the herb eases the pain and the weight of the mud in our shoes. Or really in the Adidas sneakers we peeled off this fly wacko who came to deal once. He was only a kid and went real still when we pulled the knife on him and said, "Hand over the sneakers, punk," and then your jeans and your shirt. And just to be nice we didn't flatten his nose, since his teeth were chattering. And even though he was flush we felt sorry for him and counted to ten, same as the cops count for us, we did the same thing for that kid, because here we are the law, this is our turf, though all the old ladies yell at us and keep mopping the stairs so we can't sit down. So we go to the housing blocks round back and suddenly the corner's empty because the cops show up and the running starts and the beatings, they even force their way into the apartments, dragging us to the curb and then down to the slammer. And though we're clean they charge us just the same and your old lady has to somehow find the money to pay the fine and I'm promising her never again, that I'll find a job and earn lots of money so we can leave the projects. Because she lives with her heart in her hands when I don't come home. And though I tell her she can relax she no longer believes me and keeps shouting it's twelve, get out of bed, when for me the only twelve is midnight, when there's a party waiting for me on a Friday or Saturday, waiting for me to die one of these days for being alive as I am.

The bodies of these shantytown juniors keep stockpiling the city cemetery week after week. And if you can't afford a grave, there's the cemetery's wall of shelves, which looks just like the projects, re-creating poverty's quarters for eternity.

It would seem that said file-cabinet urbanism was designed to underscore the confusion and madness of life for the marginalized, via the city's distribution of space and through force of human accumulation, as if life was not already violent enough.

It would seem, then, that every birth in one of these housing blocks, every undulating diaper announcing a new life must be stained by a tragic future. Detergents and their advertising's cheerful sunshine seem useless; scrubbing is useless; professional or university dreams are useless for these kiddos in the back row. Forgotten by teachers inside the city bureaucracies that redline education according to neighborhood and the status of its inhabitants. Neoliberal inheritance or future capitalist boom in this absurd demo of a democracy. An unreachable future for these kids, just the cruel joke of candidacy, a free society's betrayal. Saving them from army boots just to have them end up as jerky smoked on the same carcass, on the same wreck where they were born. What a horizon for this stratum of young people who gambled their best years. Already beyond hope, already heaped together in modernity's crepuscular underclass. Light-years away from the million-dollar tuitions the rich shell out for their saplings at private institutions.

Already cannon fodder in the scuffles of big politics. In the shadows to snort, rob, fuck—if there's already nothing to lose, and any day now he could be found with his ribs up in the air. Surely understandable tactics for surviving these new Middle Ages. A way to refuse political mockery and the hit-and-runs of the law. An uncertain future for these kids exposed to crime, who cast as South America's castoffs couldn't make ends meet. Irredeemably lost to the projects' apocalyptic journey. . . . sailing calmly through social utopia's urban decay.

THE ABYSS OF SOUND

Outside of Trujillo, in Peru, you can find what remains of Chan Chan, a pre-Incan city that sleeps in ruins worn smooth by the ocean breeze. Everything's made out of mud, which, despite being fragile, radiates a brilliant reddish brown and warms the adobe with the same color as Indigenous skin. The main square is a huge rectangle at the muddied metropolis's center: a wall runs along the periphery, covered in reliefs of fish swimming in opposite directions. There's a point where the shoals come together, crisscrossing. It lines up with the Humboldt Current, which crosses right at Trujillo, mixing northern waters with the frigid southern sea.

Tourists and couples have scrawled names, dates, slogans, and doodles on this clay wall, imposing Spanish writing on top of its zoomorphic alphabet, which, in its simplicity, in its flash of fishes and the harsh murmur of the Pacific, maps the whole salty horizon.

But beyond any theories that make the magic of these hieroglyphs correspond to modern science, as signs they speak another language, hard to translate into writing's logic. Maybe they're not concepts that linear thought has arranged but drawings that hold noises, voices pressed into the mud, guttural descriptions of a pre-Columbian geography whose elements dazzled the white man with the music of color. Meaning these shapes might also be translated as a humming repository of syllables, or as scores for the lively music of a Mesoamerican earthquake. For the speech and laughter in the murmurous thumping of the Andean heart. For the shared and mourned as the blood crashes through arterial promontories. A voice that mimics the surroundings, like a mockingbird who traces a looping call between the trees. Until writing came and, with it, the Spanish alphabet that stifled her song.

These aural networks raised a cry to warn tribes of the coming invasion. The sound of waves could be heard in high plateaus through conches and seashell trumpets, the mollusk species that raised the alarm across all of Tawantinsuyu. Just like the cries of birds when a hunter's boot crushes the weeds. Or the closed-lip murmur that now passes between Indian women at border checkpoints. Inexact syllables that put the officer who lets them through on edge with their smuggled chitchat. Like parrots chittering in half tongues, that call of *puis-puis-puis*, untranslatable to the page, to the written word, so foundational, so orderly, so universal—so brimming with thought, our feverish Western minds. Our solipsism in thinking that memories are stored in mute libraries, where the only thing that echoes is the word SILENCE printed on a plaque.

But that *chsss* is not silence—for an Indigenous tongue, *chsss* might have something to do with a toothache, and the *s* is the fan that cools the burning molar. Maybe *chsss* is also the shish of rain on straw roofs or a snake's hiss while laying eggs in the tall grass. How to translate this? How to teach our haughty brains all the meaning a sound carries?

The logic of the alphabet holds us prisoner. Our upbringing leads us down a path in our minds that the ABCs illuminate for us. But just past the edge of the page is an abyss where there are no letters. A jungle full of noises, like a secret market with scents and flavors and strange words that keep changing meaning. Words that gain color only once they're in the receiver's heart. Sounds that hide in the corner of the mouth to remain beneath writing's notice.

Just past the edge of the page you're reading burbles a Babel of foulmouthed, unreadable voices, always giving the slip to any definitions that literature has sussed out of them.

Supposedly, the page contains both a voice and the desire that voice expresses. This belief, however, assumes that proper, Catholic writing always existed in the Americas. Between two letters is a confession; between two words, a commandment.

What is read is read to us before the eyes of God. The sacred texts bear his signature. The Incan emperor Atahualpa didn't know this, which is why he mistook the Bible for a conch shell, and placed it against his ear to hear the creator's words aloud. But that black and rectangular shell didn't hold the hush of the mountains or the echoes of the sea. Hearing nothing, Atahualpa threw the Bible on the ground and gave Friar Vicente de Valverde a pretext for justifying the Conquest's genocide. The Incan also didn't know that, years later, the Catholic king Carlos II would outlaw the use of any native tongues. Atahualpa had died before learning to read, and, illiterate, he kept listening beneath the earth to the sound of the tides like an endless language.

Perhaps writing as a mechanism can't be undone, and our literate memory is written culture's triumph, together with Pizarro's, over Atahualpa's aural world. But this only shows us that reading and writing are more instruments of power than of thought. And maybe the scar of a letter imprinted on memory can still open in the shape of an O, a mouth for swallowing a gag whole. Domitila's testimony in *Let Me Speak!*, first published in 1977, shows us this is possible, as well as Felipe Huamán Poma de Ayala's chronicles, finished in 1615. These and other texts are examples of how orality can use writing, dubbing over its domain while at the same time appropriating freely from it.

There are many kinds of silences that scriptured culture imposes on colonized oral ethnicities, but learning to read those silences is to relearn to speak. To use what words omit, deny, or fabricate, so that we know what's hidden from us, what's not said or understood. That silence is ours, but it is not silence. It speaks like a memory exorcising its colonial stamp and piecing together an oral dignity that the alphabet destroyed.

CENSUS AND THE CONQUEST

(. . . AND THAT PINK WIG UNDER THE BED?)

One of the first censuses in the Americas was undertaken by the Catholic Church during the Conquest. While the colonizing armies were busy massacring indigenous towns and villages, the Jesuits went around knocking on doors, noting anything that might give Native Americans an advantage over the Spanish. The foreigners dismembering the New World's features into a profile marred by statistics, eager to classify the pre-Columbian mystery into logical statutes and stratifications of power.

Before Europe plunged in its sword with its bloody horror-scope, pre-Hispanic cosmology had relied on other measurements. The stone calendars rotated in cycles of spinning expansion and return, analogously tied to periods of fertility, dryness, or rest.

Time depended on other parameters, having more to do with a revolving wheel than quantitative numbers. The indigenous didn't know how to respond to these clerical questions, vested in dominance and a certain morbid white curiosity. How much coitus per week? How many masturbations per month, on average? How do so many of you live in a single hut? How many mortal sins can be added to the rosary's glass accounting? How many prayers and Hail Marys do they recite to be absolved? How many square feet of gold would they pay as tribute? Facing an avalanche of harassment, the indigenous responded without any of the math of the original questions, as it felt more like being accused, having confessed to living on their own land with practices from their own environment. Just to say something, they replied four or four hundred, from shaping their lips to make "our." They said a million for the way the tongue chimed, fluttering like a strange insect on the roof of the mouth. They chose five for the whistling of air as it crossed broken teeth, murmured six for the rain's generous whisper on their straw roofs. The number's sound switched for quantifiable meaning, for the oral relationship between a question and the act of response. Sidestepping elliptically the survey's unofficial agenda, escaping the appeals by appearing to be idiots, which threw off the missionaries' Gothic calculus. The indigenous used the ancient art of camouflage to defend themselves, disturbing the rigid numeric symbols with the semiotics of their surroundings.

The results of the census and surveys were delivered to European bourgeois society, describing the immoral and promiscuous lives of America's inhabitants. The church and the monarchy declared them savage, inspiring future voyages of discovery with an evangelizing spirit. For this many heretics, so many sabers; for this many animals, so many cages.

Hundreds of years later, we are again facing a population census that wants to tally up citizen habits, supposedly so they can adjust the amount of shortfall in our developing economy. Once again the social worker's empty suit will make her grand visit will seat herself on the edge of a chair. And shooing away the flies she'll wet her lips with discolored tea from the only teacup that still has a handle. Asking how many beds, how many are working—and those who aren't, what do they do? And the teenage daughter who's waiting behind the curtain for the señorita to leave so she won't see the streetwalker's purple shadow under her eyes. And the pink wig the mother hides as she lets the señorita into the room of her son who works up north. Rattling off the wonderful presents he sends her from Iquique as she discreetly shoves a pair of high heels under the bed. Demonstrating how the double cassette radio works, and the color TV. Pulling out a string of tchotchkes she'll never use, too worried about getting them dirty. The mother who strokes the silver insignia of a refrigerator empty of things to eat but pregnant with little cubes of ice.

Like an anteater, the super-census sticks its trunk into poverty's grimy folds while its official pen makes an inventory of each household's instability. If the walls are cement or mud mixed with straw. If they have a toilet or just a latrine. And if a toilet, then why is the water overflowing with geraniums like some Greco-Roman pot in the garden. And if the house came with a stove, why are they using it as a nightstand and making their fires with wood. And why even with so much information are the babies multiplying like rabbits. And the pets, the dogs and cats—where in the survey are they counted, because children and animals can get mixed up under the same coat of tar, the same perspiring rag that blankets misery. The curtain that the mother draws while her hand is beneath her apron, covering up a bag of marijuana, the hustle of her younger son who's doing so well working with an uncle they don't know but who buys him Adidas sneakers and always drops him off in a car. The other half of the family budget, the census negative where there's no checkbox, wearing an innocent look for any censuring eye. Waterfalls of tears sometimes even pour forth while telling the visitor the whole sad tango. You have to put on your worst clothes, get ahold of three screaming babies, and surround yourself with flies like velvet ropes at the movies just to avoid getting tangled in the bureaucracy of government assistance.

This is one way that minorities make their trafficked existence viable, outsmarting the pious enumeration of their defects. The printed list of necessities the census unfolds over Chile, like a computational snake that swallows the population's economic indexes, in order to digest them in a way that agrees with the gastro-political system. Figures and percentages will fill the mouths of every member of parliament, listing the spending numbers through the mutual fondling of partisan debate. The skinny Chilean intestine x-rayed and exposed at its best neoliberal angle like some kind of development orthopedics. A sociological sketch that does not translate in its most finely split hairs, that traces its thick lines of calculus across the underbelly that sustains the political class, across the undocumented interconnections that go spoiling democracy's project of self-determination.

Maybe an inheritance that surfaces within the margins as a containment strategy when facing recolonialization via paperwork. Maybe a micropolitics of survival that works from within the subtext of their lives, palming off the mechanisms of government control. An undoing that smiles at the census bureau and says goodbye at a door made of wooden boards with an expression that perfectly imitates politeness, with a traitorous see you later that fills every column with zero, like a tribal pre-language that hermetically closes the seal of disobedience.

YOU'RE MINE, GIRL

It was nearly dawn when I stumbled over him, wrong side of the Alameda, skirting the gutter of a yawn. He was stooped on the ground, looking for half-used cigarettes, the filters that smokers toss aside when they get on the bus. He was clearly a hip-hop kid, the wide waistband of his jeans dancing low on his narrow hips. A sapling on stick-skinny legs finished off with trusty sneakers, no laces, no ties, the way first-timers wear them in jail. Those eighteen-wheeler sneakers that boys adore like their girlfriends, their darling sneakers that they treat like an extra pair of feet, the streetwise scaffolding that transports them over the sidewalks voodooing la city. We ran into each other like that, distrust hitting us all of a sudden with its freezing metal. Want a cigarette? I surprised him, holding out a pack that he quickly snatched from me. What are you up to at this time of night? I said offhand, watching as the sunrise outlined the back of the cordillera. Just here, cold as shit, looking for a bit of cash and a warm little bed, he muttered, dispersing the smoke with a numb exhale. How much? For what? He asked, lowering his shaved head, where an NY bandana crowned his illusions. To sleep with me, I raised my voice, stressing how fragile it is to be the one who pays. Are you good with ten? That's a lot, I'll give you five and a place to stay. What do you mean? Just like la Señora Sota's boardinghouse—bed, breakfast, and tush to boot. Then he laughed harder than anything. Something my grandmother used to say, I throw out, more confident. Let's go, then . . .

And so off we went, side by side in search of a bottle to butter us up for the rubdown. What do you drink? With this cold, anything that burns. But my friends and I don't really drink; a sweet little joint and we sway with the music, the graffiti, the vibe, brother. You got music at your place? Of course, there's always music at my knackered house, but no rap or hip-hop, maybe a Los Temerarios album that I put on when the silence smothers me. That's okay, he said, opening his backpack, I've got plenty of rap on cassettes, we can sway to these. Then I realized this was no brief encounter; the kid was planning to move in, while I was looking only for a dusty passenger. But anyway . . . there we were, going to slaughter, walking past buildings scrawled with graffiti grammar and its anarchic outlines. Those are sticks, see it says: I'm the greatest and I don't back down, signed Kid Bronx. Look, over there, written by Fredy: My color is music. But I can't understand anything, I just see lines. How do you read what it says? You have to get each letter, look, see how this is a reverse *S* that can become a *Z*. Do you have pen and paper? Yes, at home. Then I'll teach you. But once we got there, the only thing I was interested in was his goldfinch body bundled in the enormous clothes of his rapper aesthetic. He shivered on the edge of the bed when he took off his sweatshirt. I'm skinny everywhere, he said, touching his ribs. What happened to your shoulder? I asked, coming closer to touch the rope of a violent scar. It was a mad fall . . . looks ugly, right? No. But how did it happen? It was at a skate meetup. I'd never gotten on that crap, but they wigged me out . . . like, don't think you're so great if you're too chicken to get on, dummy, like I'm just a wuss. And so that's why I did it, and that's why I wanted to do the craziest spin, and that's why I ate shit and a half when I jumped over the railing thinking I was a pro surfer. But up there I suddenly got that it wasn't so easy when my foot slipped and I fell ten feet down onto cement stairs. Man, the sound was hollow. I shoved my shoulder back and you could see the bone, and the pain . . . I can't even explain it, I blacked out and woke up three days later already sewn up in a fancy-ass clinic. And who paid for it all? It cost two million, brother, two million that my old lady didn't have anywhere, you feel me? And? We didn't know what to do, my old lady in that hospital room all day ragging on me, saying it was my fault, if I weren't so crazy this wouldn't have happened, how are we going to pay now and shit like that. And then? I told her I wouldn't fuck around anymore and that I'd get us out of there somehow. And one moonless night, like in the song, she tiptoed in with my clothes and helped me get dressed in the dark. There wasn't anyone in the hallways, and no one asked us where we were going either, if they'd have stopped us we would've told them we were from cleaning, because we were carrying a bucket and mop. We had it all planned out. We didn't pay shit—where would it have come from? If my old lady barely earns enough to eat selling crap at the flea market. Your mom's brave, I murmured, touched. When she wakes up on the right side of the bed, she's amazing, but she's always tired and that's why I want to help out. How? With the ten pesos I'm getting from you. The deal was five and nothing more, I said curtly. Nothing more, so little for this pretty thing? He added with his harlot eyes as he slid his hand down his tight torso and beneath his waistband until he was holding his critter in a proud fist. Touch it, I won't tell, he insisted, rowing under his pants. But he was so thin with his fraying twenty-something corporality, practically a sprig of parsley tossed into my bed, asking me to put a price on his sprouted bud. And I did, but held my breath and felt my anus cringe in terror when I touched that monster. It's the only thing I have a lot of, he stammered with sadness. It looks like a submarine torpedo, I said, excited, using both my hands to grasp the plaything with its purple head. Give it a kiss, to make it laugh. And with this same mouth that sings Ave Maria I grazed that pink peach with its hairless flowering mallow, just barely pressed my lips to that living flesh made of dry skin, little pulsating veins that pumped the leathery rind of that huge juicy mango until it almost burst. The boy twisted, growling: Ay, that feels so good, brother. That's great, man. Keep going just like that, with a mic, easy now, with a ska rhythm, like a DJ, rap to me, as if it were rap, sample me all over, son of a bitch. Yes, a little lower, hip-hopped, by the nuts, sloop-sloop-sloop . . . sloop-sloop-sloop . . . sloop-sloop-slap.

I didn't know much about hip-hop culture, maybe just what

any passerby knows from looking at the street corners where boys show off their New York style and high-five to say hello, spinning on the ground to a rhythm's improvised beats. The hip-hop wave took off among our nation's punksters a little while back, arriving with the now-retro music video. And you can see those videos imitated here, since the pubescent teens feel seen in their baggy clothing and that arrogance of being, that life-giving audacity that Black and anarchist punksters flaunt in Yanquiparadise. What's more, that speak-singing declaring punk dignity seemed to revive the rebellious glory and socio-economic alarm bells of discontent. The tall and discolored buildings in the Bronx, their lyrical lumpen tingling was a back-drop that our faded housing projects could reproduce. Almost everything was there: their unemployed leisure time exposing their minimal lives, their aspirations for the future drifting without a future in the plaza's inhospitable ring, wanting to look fashionable, which is natural even if advertisements are what's casting the particular spell, brand jeans, that blue dream that keeps the punk awake at night but vanishes into gray when his laborer's pay won't cut it, the police raid that grabs him loitering and before he goes into the cell they take the laces from his sneakers so he has to walk flopping like a clown, they snatch his belt, too, and his jeans fall down, slide right over his skinny waist, halfway past his ass, revealing the waistband of a pair of cheap briefs. So in Harlem and the Bronx the youth began wearing their pants low on their hips and their sneakers untied in solidarity with those who've been detained in police raids . . . In short, so much to say, so much to denounce, so much to sing, not knowing how to sing, con-fessioned the boy to me that morning in my house, post-fellatio. Because our music is about denouncing, brother, he said, swallowing the smoke from his cigarette. And there aren't any love songs? I suggested romanticoyly, spitting out a pubic hair twisted around my tongue. Not really, don't be so gay about it. I'm hungry, you got something to eat?

Before heading out, he scarfed down the only piece of stale bread that the rats hadn't touched, and I listened to him hum a musical phrase that he accompanied with snapping fingers.

Then he pulled out of his backpack an arsenal of cassettes, which he put on the stereo. And that was when the rap concert nightmare began. Listen, this is French rap, he said, dancing and singing, while I watched his symmetrical twisting in a trance, my mouth hanging open. Like my music, bi-boy? Yeah, I sighed, getting swept up in his rebellious energy. The stretchy to-and-fro of his breakdancing made him look like a broken doll. I won't charge you for the show, I'll give it to you for free. It's easy, wanna learn? I don't think I could, I'm already getting old, I don't dance anymore . . . you dance for me, I added, a bit shy. Heeeeey, ah ah aah, I don't think this part's gonna dance for you, he smiled, touching himself between the legs, hard again. I accepted the challenge with audacity: Let's see if I can. And he threw himself into bed, stripping with emergency quickness. He was a three-legged mosquito, moving his pelvis to the beat of the city's buzzing rhythms. Come here, sucker, don't be afraid, I'll be real careful, he said, his tense obelisk summoning me to the rite. Not that I played hard to get. I'm not scared, I'm not scared, I've seen worse, I repeated to give me courage while he slid the condom on. But the huge rammer made me gasp anyway. Oof, my eyeballs almost popped out of their sockets. Take it out, take it out, you're destroying me, I begged. Lie still, that's it, lie still, he said, gripping me tight. Relax, it's almost over, it only hurts right at first. And he was right, one carnal thrust and then his stick figure was surfing my anal runway. See that? he repeated, slobbering in my ear, it was just like that at first. Like that, just like that, breathe my brother, he whispered, raising and lowering his hips and repeating: a bit further, little cocksucker. Easy now, move nice and easy, easy like that, my boy, girl, you're mine. You're mine, girl, I thought I heard him say in his panting's passionate collage. That sounds like a rap lyric, I said, interrupting the focused rocking. But he couldn't hear me anymore, he was in ecstasy, his electric pricker machine-gunning me with its semen waterfall.

Let's put on some music, he petitioned, hissing as he reached for a cigarette. You're mine, girl, you said a little while ago, I murmured, turning on the stereo. I said that? Yes, you said that, and it sounds like a rap lyric. Wait, don't put on music. Pass me some paper and a pencil, he ordered, with a musical grin. Let's write a song, bi-boy, I'll give it to you for free. And like that, both of us strewn across the bed, he'd throw out a phrase and I'd respond with another line. This was what we came up with:

You're mine, girl
You pay for what's in me
Now don't go baking cakes, brother
I ain't no Walt Disney
You're mine, girl
If you pay me I'll be yours
It's all I have to give, brother
A cock that hurts like love
You're mine, girl
But night can make me easy
At five you didn't show, brother
At six the rubber's gone
You're mine, girl
I'm slipping from your bed
A new man will find you soon, brother
Some other strange jokester.

No one ever wrote me a song before: ingenious, obscene, not much to it, but the kid had put his feelings into those lyrics. Then he told me he would lay some music on top of it. Why bother? I said, if while you sing I can accompany you with my beatbox suck of sloop-sloop-sloop, sloop-sloop-slap.

That turned into days of rapping, drumming, scheming, drinking, and smoking spliffs up to our ears. Music would be playing no matter what time it was, and I even got used to its insistent cardiac tum-tum, it began to seem essential on the nights when his baby stud body was like a cussword worn out by our struggle between the sheets. I'd never before spent a week straight Monday to Saturday in the afternoon delights of a juicy skewering. Never before, I swear, and after giving him so much anal cumbia and merengue, I began to stay cavernously and stereophonically open. A fart was just a note in the cathedral harmony, the raucous and hollow meowing of a symphonic opera where the trombone's nighttime solo would huff and puff some hullabaloo from 1812 . . . at full floozy blast. I ended up so wide, so vacant, like someone had swung the backyard door open; a draft came in from behind, a cold wind that whirled inside my spiraled tar-paper garage. With pure rap, papi, with pure toots, I put up a fight for the baby raptor. And apparently I didn't do so bad in the orchestra exam, because when I asked him, What score do I get? the punk, sucking his cigarette greedily, said, A six and a half. That's all? I said, irritated. Seven is for the ladies, brother. He practically had it all: a piping-hot bum, bed, bread, beer, and marijuana; but an Eve howling at night would leave him restless, he'd want to go out, find girls, smell the fresh air of a conch shell. I'll come see you after, he'd say . . . And the hours would go by, back to the silence of an old, bored faggot looking out the window . . . and then he would appear again, glowing, decorated with new scars the street had awarded him. I wanted to love him, but at the same time I held back . . . but I did feel happy . . . no, it was something deeper. One day he showed up with his sneakers falling apart, shouting: I can't go around like this. A pair of these costs at least a hundred dollars, brother. Don't worry, I have glue, I'll fix them for you, I said. And in the blink of an eye I took them off him and quickly repaired his sneakers like some Christmas fairy. He just sat there surprised, his mouth open, having to swallow his consumerist anxieties. But on the days when I woke up a generous sated carnivorous rose, I showered him with gifts, enflowered him with clothing. Ten bucks at a secondhand clothing store could make him look like an elegant dandy from the Bronx. And just like that we'd stroll around Gay Town, crooning our improvised tunes. I almost got used to his freshness of living, laughing, and fucking without any of the usual cheap drama. Everything was going so well, couldn't ask for better, but eventually either he or I couldn't stand the nuptial show any longer.

I'll be right back, he said like always, and I let him go, knowing that freedom was the punk's suitcase, his most precious belonging. One night went by, then more nights, a week, but he never appeared again on my street corner. Some part of him loved me, the homeless rapper who'd lodged in my heart. But some kind of bourgeois gay shacking-up could be seen coming, and that future frightened both of us. Which is why, after a period of waiting like Penelope, I put away his rap lyrics and graffiti sketches and returned to the insomnia of the faggot foxes' alleyways. And that's where I am now, half in darkness, like a graying bitch, sniffing each pissed-on corner in case the air's rose garden contains a whiff of his swaying, wounded steps.

THE TRANSFIGURATION OF MIGUEL ÁNGEL

(OR, "FAITH MOVES MOUNTAINS")

Every so often in Chile—and this depends on the day's politics, as the opportunistic news media will spread or squash local events accordingly—the Virgin Mary appears in the bark of trees, in the peeling paint of an abandoned mural, in a whorehouse's broken window, in a chicken coop where birds lay eggs imprinted with Our Lady's face, in Pinochet's bullet-splintered car windshield, in Coca-Cola bottle caps, in a sports team's tattered flag, in short, just about everywhere, without warning, the Mother of Christ reenacts her glowing performance to the first person who sees her, leaving him with his eyes rolled back, certified as a healer for being the one chosen to tune into sainthood TV.

Such was the notorious case of Miguel Ángel from Villa Alemana. The child saint, the pubescent medium who overnight traded his miserable life at an orphanage for fame as a miracle-worker who could speak to the Virgin face-to-face. Before that afternoon, Miguel Ángel was just another Chilean little boy who forgot to scrub behind his ears. And his town hadn't been in the news since the earthquake. So no one imagined that this poor urchin would be the one to start such a ruckus, repeating I saw her, I saw her, she spoke to me. And the whole town poured out to see it, with the mayor, the priest, the teachers, the firemen, and busybodies all running, all trampling each other to reach the hill where the kid said the Virgin was waiting for him. Right there, on those crags, on that mount, there's a lady in white calling me. You don't see her? She's so pretty. Look how she smiles at me. But no one saw anything but rocks and brambles. No one can see her because the Immaculate doesn't want us to, one woman said. She only shows herself to children who are pure, and in this town the people are lousy and fight too much. Miguel Ángel is the only one she's let in, to delight himself in her brightness. And this seemed to be true, because when the hour of his meeting with the Lady of the Dawn arrived, Miguel Ángel entered a state of ecstasy. And his raving meditation meant that the whole crowd became participants in his miracle as they watched him fall to the ground, his face like a spaced-out archangel, praying in tongue twisters and foreign phrases that the pious among them identified as Latin and Mapuche.

The throng of people who'd followed the kid burst into sobs and mea culpas when the shakes overtook him, those attacks, that epilepsy of the spirit twisting and turning him on the rocks as he clawed at his face, tore his hair out in fistfuls. They couldn't hold him down, he was as strong as a bull, even five men couldn't constrain him. He was banged up all over, because the world has become so wicked, said the women. Because so many terrible things happen here in this country, the poor thing's turned into a child Christ who pays for our sins.

So the news of Villa Alemana's Boy Who Cried Mary spread beyond the usual boundaries of farm-country gossip, especially once it got around that a cripple had taken off running, a blind man said he could see the American flag on the moon, and a mute got a job as a sports broadcaster on the radio. That's when the pilgrimages started—the crowds of sick seeking a cure, and the healthy but bored who wanted to contract the epidemic of faith. Paralytics arrived by the truckload; the lame and syphilitic dragging their hernias left an oozing path on the trail. All trying to reach the healing hands of the radiant child saint, the shining Miguel Ángel, the town's very own beatitude, now comfortably settled in a house fit for a queen, where his secretaries took surveys, made initial diagnoses, handed out queue numbers, and swatted people with brooms to keep the crush of them at bay, the sick and dying who beat each other with their canes trying to get an appointment. There was such a fuss that the story soon reached Santiago. And the journalists came running, panting into their tape recorders and jotting things on their notepads. And television crews showed up with infrared cameras to record evidence of alien life, which, rumor had it, had landed in Pinochet's Chile to speak with a poor boy. So much uproar that the heads of the diocese began to worry, always wary of these bouts of popular faith. And after a number of long meetings the bishop decided to send an old rector known for his exorcisms to Peña Blanca to investigate the events.

So the appointed shrivel interviewed the town priest, did some digging into the lives of the saner half of the sick, held long conversations with Miguel Ángel, and kept his eyes glued day and night to the crags where they said the Virgin had landed. He meditated, recited the rosary backward and forward, tried to feel excited about Miguel Ángel's paraplegic high-wire act, and was even tempted to stand on his head to see how the sky looked the other way around. Just to be safe, he repented a thousand times for having been a military chaplain and given communion to maybe more than a few murderers. He ate nothing, resisting the fragrant temptation of empanadas, kebabs, and garlic fritters wafting from the street fair that had taken up residence at the foot of the impromptu sanctuary. He said nothing, not even about the circus that had turned the town into an avalanche of acrobats, jugglers, hypnotists, and gypsies hawking the Virgin's sacrosanct image. He tolerated the color posters they strung up, with photos of María hugging the kid. There was every kind of picture: the Virgin as rustic maiden, as earth mother, as punk, and even one with her in a space suit stepping off a flying saucer. He played dumb before an endless procession of ignominy, putting up with it all just to see something, to find himself face-to-face with divinity, asking her why she'd chosen this nasty scamp who'd never even received his First Communion. Why, Señora, did you appear to this heretic whelp. Why do you refuse me your presence. Me, who's spent my life in flagellations and tortures just to get a glimpse of you. Why not even a glimmer, not the tiniest jolt of that electric torment that leaves all these people with their eyes crossed. Why haven't you sent me the smallest sign in all these days of putting up with so many sinners, so many wasting homosexuals scratching their pustules right beside me.

Why, Señora? I, who have kept my eyes open and my heart in peace for a week, fasting with my mouth full of earth and my intestines all dried up. Trying to quiet my anger, straining to catch some gleam so that I might receive the smallest spark of your grace. To not leave as I came. And nothing, nada, nothing. Nothing but a sham, nothing but the sheer humbuggery of quacks and the poor. Nothing but a racket, those miracles of that Miguel Ángel. Collective suggestibility, I'll write in my report to the archbishop. And if I'm wrong, only God will know.

But the official diagnosis of the Peña Blanca case, far from discrediting Miguel Ángel's healing powers, made them all the more popular, as the many faithful who distrust the church now became his fans. His fame spread beyond national borders, bringing pilgrims from all over the world: the incurably sick, who'd already toured the big-ticket sanctuaries of Lourdes, Fátima, and Lo Vásquez; gringos sweaty with cancer; lepers from India; locas sick with evictions and AIDS who'd leave their visit in a fever of healing, thanking the Virgin for her miracle, kissing Miguel Ángel's hands, Miguel Ángel who, unmoved, accepted voluntary donations as payment for his healing powers. Gifts and travelers checks and installments paid in dollars, which was already adding up to a small fortune. To build a temple to Our Señora, Miguel Ángel would always reply, tired of the same indiscreet questions, exhausted by the same gossipy interviews, the same ritual day in and day out of kissing boo-boos better.

Which is why—and having received many invitations from abroad—he decided to take some time off. And so one day he closed up shop, explaining that he was headed to an international conference of the enlightened. And the whole town saw him off at the highway with tears in their eyes. The mayor read a long and emotional speech, and then, borne up by the applause, Miguel Ángel flew from his native land, offering blessings through the bus window until all they could see was a blue speck vanishing into the distance.

Without their saint, the town soon slid back into its anonymous languor. The wind went about dismantling the altars, and the winter rain took charge of fading any posters washed up in the storms. The shoemaker broke down his refreshment stand and returned to shoes, the seamstress put away her vials of earth from the mount and resumed sewing, the teacher had no more clients who needed divine messages translated and picked up her chalk again, and so all the young kids stopped being tour guides, hating the return to school. And then and suddenly and for a long time after, everything went back to being tragically as it was.

Years passed, and in Santiago the resistance bombarded the streets. The dictatorship watched, griping and grumbling, as the pearly airs of democracy breezed in. And so with everyone caught up in all the political changes, Miguel Ángel disappeared from memory.

When a newspaper announced that the child saint was returning to Chile, few could recall who he was. Two or three journalists showed up at the airport to wait for him, and after watching so many exiles step off the plane and, crying and slobbering, kiss the ground of their homeland, after watching them unload half of Europe as their luggage, shouting in French to a bunch of Mapuche kids who refused to leave their seats, But a-why? Chile, it eez still ahgly. I vant to goh bahk to Paris, the returning milksops pleaded, screeching in a mixture of languages as their parents dragged them out by their ears. After this display was over, when no passengers were left and the journalists, feeling duped, were hurrying to pack up. A girl with long hair and dark glasses approached them, swarmed by attendants, just like the first day she boarded a plane. Don't you recognize me? I'm Miguel Ángel. The Virgin made me a woman.

The entire country tuned in to watch the TV special about the child saint's miraculous transfiguration. To flesh out the biography portion, they dusted off their old Peña Blanca images: the crowds, the Virgin's hill, photos of the adolescent

Christ in raptures, his crystal gaze, his purity back then like a heavenly nymph—compared to this floozy with long black hair and big tits and red lips giving an exclusive interview with Canal Nacional. There wasn't much left of Miguel Ángel, angel of the sick and the lame. Just something in her voice, now hoarser with age, giving thanks to the Virgin for the transsexual lightning bolt that had changed her gender.

The program also included testimony from people who were close to her. They interviewed the elderly doctor at the orphanage, who confirmed that as a child Miguel Ángel was a big, healthy boy, with a penis and properly formed testicles. I know because I was the only one who gave him regular checkups, that I'm sure of. But now I have no idea, I'm baffled by the medical reports saying she's a woman and doesn't show any signs of surgery. He says—sorry, she says—that the Virgin offered him one last miracle, because she was weary and wanted to retire. Who knows? I'm not a believer but "faith can move mountains." Besides, there are things even science doesn't understand.

After the commercial break, a bishop spoke. He said the Blessed María didn't perform this sort of miracle, or meddle in divine creation—no matter how motherly she may be, she wasn't able to change the will of the Creator, who made man good and manly and woman, well, nice and womanly. The Bible is very clear about these things, it doesn't accept sexual operations with mystic scalpels, or sodomite tricks. The Virgin doesn't act alone, she's directed by the Almighty, who is the final word.

The controversial documentary broke all television ratings. The camera showed Miguel Ángel brushing her hair, painting her nails, ironing and cooking like a country lass. They also filmed her going for a walk on the hill where the Virgin had appeared, hand in hand with her new fiancé. A young flaming macho who declared they were going to marry as soon as possible and live happily ever after, and that their kids . . . well, the Virgin never runs out of miracles, and, as they say, faith can move mountains.

Almost everyone involved appeared in the television trial—everyone minus the elderly exorcist priest, now very old and repeating that the Virgin had finally given him proof of her grace, that, after so much pleading, María, touched, had appeared to him in the flesh through Miguel Ángel's transfiguration, and that he could now die in peace after seeing her face on TV, speaking to him. She was so pretty, so young, her merciful gaze so lovely in that photo the newspaper published, which he clipped for his altar, so he could drape her in flowers, replacing his old image of that unfashionable señora.

The old priest was one of the only people who swallowed the story, and he bid the world goodbye still ecstatic over his virgin travesti. Within the week, the rest of the country had forgotten all about the outlandish telenovela, and no more was heard from Miguel Ángel, no magical healing powers ever made the news. Surely because she didn't have time, busy with all the household chores.

Nobody in town wanted to talk about it—nobody turned on the TV or even opened the newspaper that day. A cloud of silence formed over the subject, erasing the name Miguel Ángel from the memory of everyone who lived there. The only thing left was the mount, deep in the countryside, which the moon's brightness lit up from time to time, softening the granite erection with its misty cloak. Way up there, in the middle of the night, another kind of visitor still makes the trek, camouflaged in the shadows: travesti pilgrims who climb Peña Blanca's slope, carrying their high heels in one hand. Ladybirds who want to be women, destitute transsexuals who don't have money for the operation, nudist hermaphrodites who expose their prostates to the moon, hoping for the heavenly axe. They're the only ones who still honor the sanctuary, who still irrigate its rocky crags with candles, the only ones who make rapturous vows to strike and hold a diva pose until the clatter of daybreak. To see if María hears them, up in the sky; to see if their mamita Virgen, on the sly and behind God's back, comes down to Earth to repeat her miracle—as cheap, as soft as being struck by a lily, no anesthesia and free of pain.

Notes

IN LIEU OF A SYNOPSIS

1 **the milonga drag of a travestango starlet:** Colloquially, a milonga refers to a gathering or venue where people dance tango, usually accompanied by live music.

2 **Paquita la del Barrio:** A well-known Mexican singer of ranchera-style ballads. Her stage name translates to Paquita from the Neighborhood.

MARICÓN

HER THROATY LAUGH

6 ***¿Cuánto vale el show?*:** A talent-search television show on Chilevisión, primarily in the early eighties but with reboots on and off in the nineties and the first decade of the twenty-first century.

6 **a yellow Lada:** A common car in 1980s Chile, imported from Russia.

MANIFESTO

9 **the CNI's electric grill:** the Central Nacional de Informaciones (CNI, or National Information Center). The grill (in Spanish, *parrilla*) was the name for a common form of torture in Chile, where victims would be strapped down to an old metal bed-frame that was wired with high-voltage electricity.

10 **Colo-Colo:** One of the major soccer teams in Chile.

ANACONDAS IN THE PARK

13 ***verde que te quiero verde***: "Green how I want you green." Lemebel quotes the opening line of "Romance sonámbulo," a poem by gay Spanish poet and playwright Federico García Lorca (1898–1936).

CHILE: SEA MEN AND CUECA

19 **A chilenidad:** As glossed in the first paragraph, *chilenidad* means, roughly, Chilean-ness. While Chilean folk culture and revivalism is tied to Allende and his supporters (see, for example, "Where Were You?"), the rural tropes Lemebel describes here are typical of Chilean "huaso" (or cowboy) culture, associated with Chile's big ranching estates and conservative cultural nationalism.

19 **The cueca is a dance that reenacts the Spanish conquest:** While a vision of the cueca reenacting the entire Spanish conquest is highly Lemebelian, the cueca is popularly considered to be a dance that personifies the act of sexual pursual and seduction. The two most common interpretations are that of a rooster courting a hen, or, more disturbingly—and as Lemebel alludes to—of a colonial master "seducing" a female servant.

19 **chases the china:** *China,* from the Quechua for servant or breeding animal, was the term used for young servant girls on ranching estates up through the mid-twentieth century.

19 **Temuco's night sky:** Temuco is a city in Chile and the capital of the Araucanía region, associated with the indigenous Mapuche people and their resistance to the Spanish Empire (and later to the Chilean government).

20 ***arréglate, Juana Rosa, que te llegó invitación***: "Get dressed, Juana Rosa / Your invitation's arrived." "Juana Rosa" is a famous song by the folk singer Violeta Parra, about a working-class girl who receives an invitation to a dance. The song encourages her to get dressed and go to the party, as she's now twenty-five and running the risk of becoming an old maid.

20 **the Eighteenth of September:** Chilean Independence Day (known as El Dieciocho), which is the holiday described in this crónica.

21 **cumbia's humming:** Originating in Colombia, cumbia is a genre of music that has gained popularity throughout Central and South America.

21 ***mira como va, negrito***: Potentially a creative mishearing of the classic salsa song "Oye cómo va," which goes, "*Oye cómo va, mi ritmo / bueno pa' gozar, mulata.*"

WILD DESIRE

33 **"learn the language of patriarchy in order to curse it":** Lemebel elsewhere attributes this quote to Bolivian activist Domitila Barrios de Chungara (1937–2012). For many English readers, the phrase is associated with Shakespeare's *The Tempest,* when Caliban says, "You taught me language; and my profit on't / Is, I know how to curse. The red plague rid you / For learning me your language!" The line is often referenced by twentieth-century Caribbean writers as emblematic of the postcolonial position.

34 **playing forever in our memory:** General Carlos Ibáñez del Campo was the leader of an earlier military dictatorship in Chile (1927–1931), and was later openly elected as president (1952–1958). Both were periods marked by the persecution of political dissidents and homosexuals—rumor includes death by drowning. The image of a group boarding a ship at Valparaíso may come from the 1940s, when many homosexual prisoners were taken from Santiago and sent by ship to Pisagua, a concentration camp in the north. Pinochet would later use the camp for political prisoners (see "Pisagua en Pointe").

35 **mestizaje:** A somewhat outdated term that refers, broadly, to the mixed-race heritage that defines much of Latin America.

35 **"victorious capitalism":** A phrase from Max Weber's *The Protestant Ethic and the Spirit of Capitalism.*

COUP

FOR FIVE MINUTES YOU BLOSSOM

39 **FOR FIVE MINUTES YOU BLOSSOM:** The title is a line from "Te recuerdo Amanda" ("I Remember You, Amanda"), a song by the revered folk singer Víctor Jara, who was a staunch supporter of the Allende government. The song recounts a romance

between two factory workers and the man's subsequent death fighting for an unnamed cause:

> For five minutes / Life is eternal for five minutes / The siren wails / Break is over / And walking back / You light up everything / For five minutes / You blossom / . . . He left for the mountains / He, who never hurt anyone / He left for the mountains / And in five minutes he was torn apart / The siren wails / Break is over / Many didn't come back / Not Manuel, either.

Víctor Jara was himself imprisoned and then killed in the first days of the coup, and, rather than disappearing the corpse, his body was prominently left outside the National Stadium, where other prisoners were still being held.

40 *como un perro que no me deja ni se calla*: The phrase—"like a dog that won't shut up or leave me alone"—appears in the poem "Umbrío por la pena," by Spanish writer Miguel Hernández, who spoke out against fascism in his poetry and died during the Spanish Civil War. Lemebel likely first heard the line in a song by the popular Catalonian singer Serrat, who recorded a 1972 album where he set Hernández's poems to music.

IF YOU DON'T RETURN

47 ***Pues la ciudad sin ti . . . está solitaria***: "Well, the city without you . . . is a lonely place." The lyrics quoted throughout come from a 1960s hit song by the Italian singer Mina. The original Italian recording is "Città vuota" (1963), and Mina also released a version of the song in Spanish as "Ciudad solitaria" ("Lonely City"), which is the version of the recording that Lemebel hears.

47 ***Todas las calles llenas de gente están, y por el aire suena una música***: "All the streets are full of people, and music trails through the air."

48 ***De noche salgo con alguien a bailar, nos abrazamos, llenos de felicidad . . . mas la ciudad sin ti . . .*** : "At night someone takes me dancing, we hold each other tight, full of happiness . . . yet the city without you . . ."

48 **Don Francisco:** The stage name of Mario Luis Kreutzberger Blumenfeld, host of *Sábados gigantes,* a long-running televi-

sion variety show in Chile (1962–1992) and later in the US (where the show's name changed slightly, to *Sábado gigante*).

MERCI, BEAU COUP

51 **strung from the cordillera:** The cordillera are the Andes. Making up a large percentage of Chile's land mass, the series of mountain ranges form a constant backdrop for the country's landscape and also isolate Chile from much of the rest of the world.

52 **she parodied Eva Perón:** Eva Perón (1919–1952) was married to Juan Perón, president of Argentina from 1946 to 1955, whose economic vision (Peronism) continues to be a major political force in Argentina. To her supporters, Eva Perón was a philanthropist, generous with the poor and constantly soliciting contributions for her welfare projects; to her detractors, Eva Perón was an ex–radio actress with expensive taste and a porous relationship to national funds.

BLACK ORCHIDS

55 **DINA'S:** Dirección de Inteligencia Nacional (National Intelligence Directorate) was the secret police of Chile, formed shortly after the coup and responsible for many of the disappearances. The agency was dissolved in 1977 and turned into the Central Nacional de Informaciones (CNI, or National Information Center).

55 **the Patria y Libertad quagmire:** See the introduction.

WHERE WERE YOU?

59 **dead ringers for Bolocco:** Cecilia Bolocco (b. 1965), a Chilean actress and beauty queen who won Miss Universe in 1987.

60 **Maluenda cheer on the armed forces on daytime TV:** Enrique Maluenda was a Chilean television host in the 1970s and 1980s.

60 **with Canto Nuevo in the canteens:** An outgrowth of the Nueva Canción music that defined the 1960s and early '70s in Chile. As much of the Nueva Canción repertoire was outlawed under Pinochet, Canto Nuevo emerged in its stead, with highly allegorical lyrics to evade censorship.

FLASH ART POLITICS: THREE TALES

71 **El Coordinador Cultural was born:** A group founded in 1983 that grew out of the Unión Nacional Por la Cultura (National Union for Culture, founded 1977).

71 **I think it must have been for September 11:** September 11, 1973, was the day the military took control of Chile. During the dictatorship, the government celebrated this day as a holiday, while activists often organized protests.

75 **the art activism that emerged from that decade:** Lemebel seems to be arguing here that the El Coordinador Cultural was a contemporary of—or even preceded—better-known groups like Colectivo Acciones de Arte (Art Action Collective, or CADA), whose members included figures like Raúl Zurita and Diamela Eltit.

76 **someone from MIR:** See the introduction. The Movimiento de Izquierda Revolucionaria (Revolutionary Left Movement) was a communist group founded in 1965. They were known for armed resistance to the dictatorship.

AIDS

DIAMONDS ARE FOREVER

84 **Like AZT:** AZT was the first antiretroviral therapy for AIDS, developed by Burroughs Wellcome and rushed to market in 1987. The drug had severe side effects and its results for a patient were temporary, as it ultimately led to the body forming AZT-resistant strains.

NIGHT OF FURS

87 **the UNCTAD building:** Created for the third United Nations Conference on Trade and Development, hosted in Santiago, Chile. The building was famously completed in nine months and with thousands of volunteers in order to be ready for the September 1972 conference.

87 **the latest episode of *Música libre*:** *Música libre* (1971–1975) was a Chilean popular music and dance television show in the style of *American Bandstand* or *Soul Train*.

88 **La Vega:** La Vega, or La Vega Central, is a legendary produce market in Santiago and looms large in the popular imagination.

88 **the Recoleta locas:** Recoleta is a working-class neighborhood in Santiago.

88 **the Blue Ballet locas, the locas from Carlina's:** Lemebel writes elsewhere about Aunt Carlina's salon and the associated Blue Ballet, a popular troupe of travesti showgirls.

88 **cruised along Huérfanos:** A street in the downtown district.

88 **Coppelia queens:** Coppelia is a café and ice cream parlor in the Providencia neighborhood. The café was particularly known in the late sixties and early seventies as a popular locale for artists, intellectuals, and students.

89 **La Astaburuaga, la Zañartu, and la Pilola Alessandri:** All these last names would be familiar to Chilean readers as denoting high-society and political families. Jorge Alessandri, for example, was president of Chile from 1958 to 1964.

93 **Kaposi's serum:** An allusion to Kaposi Sarcoma, a skin cancer that causes large purple lesions to form across the body. Once a very rare condition, developing the lesions quickly became a telltale sign of having AIDS.

93 **its Black Orpheus:** A 1959 classic of Brazilian cinema, which sets the Greek myth of Orpheus and Eurydice during Carnaval in midcentury Rio de Janeiro.

96 **shining on San Camilo Street:** Known as an area where travestis rent rooms and usually make their money from sex work.

96 **Vivaceta and Maipú and in La Sota de Talca:** Vivaceta and Maipú are streets on the northern and southern edges of Santiago, respectively. La Sota refers to the red-light district in Talca, a small city a few hours south of the capital.

96 ***que me voy bien pagá*:** A reference to "La bien pagá," sung by Miguel de Molina in the 1952 film *Ésta es mi vida*. The song is about a man ending a relationship with a prostitute—and "bien pagá" refers to the fact that she's been "well paid" for her services.

97 **a flag, with its victorious rainbow:** Lemebel is referring to the voting campaign's flag, which was white with a rainbow in the center.

THE DEATH OF MADONNA

103 **the sight of the Yeguas del Apocalipsis:** Pedro Lemebel's and Francisco Casas's performance art duo. See the introduction.

103 **cast themselves in Chinese theater:** This may be a reference either to Grauman's Chinese Theatre in Hollywood or to "Manolita Chen's Chinese Theater," a vaudeville troupe in Spain active from 1950 to 1986, run by Chen Tse-Ping and starring his wife, Manuela Fernández Pérez. Another stage performer, Manuela Saborido Muñoz, who was trans, adopted the same name—Manolita Chen—and starred in a show that competed with the Chens' on the traveling theater circuit. The professional confusion and gender ambiguity led to a tabloid scandal in Spain.

108 **that original movie poster:** Lemebel is referring to *Desperately Seeking Susan* (1985).

REGINE, QUEEN OF MONKEY ALUMINUMS

117 ***como si fuera esta noche la última vez*:** Part of the opening line of one of the iconic twentieth-century Latin American boleros, "Bésame mucho," by Mexican composer and singer Consuelo Velázquez, where she intones her lover to kiss her "as if tonight were the last time."

118 ***En vano quieres matar mi orgullo. No has visto ni verás llanto en mis ojos*:** A line from the Chilean singer Palmenia Pizarro's waltz "En vano"—"In vain you try to kill my pride / But you'll never see desperation in my eyes."

118 ***Y dicen que le hace pero no le hace, tan chiquitita y quiere casarse*:** Lyrics from a traditional Chilean tonada, "La pollita," which describes—at least on the surface—waiting for a chicken to lay an egg. "I've gotten myself for raising / a little chick in my house / she spends the day singing and singing / and she still, and she still won't lay / And they say that she will but she doesn't / so young but she wants to get married."

POST-90

FROU-FROU EXILES

142 **the Inti:** Shorthand for the Inti-Illimani, a famous Nueva Canción musical group in Chile. They were on tour in Italy when the military staged the coup, and remained there.

142 **Charo's frou-frou ribs:** Likely Charo Cofré, an exiled singer and part of the Nueva Canción movement.

142 **"Cuando me acuerdo de mi país":** "When I Remember My Country." A 1965 song by Chilean singer-songwriter Patricio Manns, who lived in exile in France during the dictatorship.

143 **peñas:** Associated with the folk revival and grassroots politics of the 1960s and early '70s, a *peña* is a small cultural center that stages performances and serves as an informal community gathering space.

143 **whiskquierda's:** A Lemebelian portmanteau of whisky and izquierda (meaning Left).

THE BALLAD OF WILLY ODDÓ

145 **a lead singer of Quilapayún:** A major music group from the Nueva Canción era. Víctor Jara served as their artistic director. Individual members of the group, including Willy Oddó, fled to Europe after the coup.

145 **revolutionary Nueva Canción music:** See the introduction.

146 **"Plegaria a un labrador":** "Prayer to a Laborer," an iconic political anthem in Chile from 1970, sung by the band Quilapayún and written by Víctor Jara, the band's artistic director during the Allende years.

146 **chant of *el pueblo unido jamás será vencido*:** A famous protest chant in Spanish, which now appears in protests around the world. It translates to "The people, united, will never be defeated."

146 **Little Luchín's same muddy bum:** A reference to "Luchín," a song by Víctor Jara about a poor boy playing outside. Lemebel's line about the boy's muddy bum is a direct quote from the lyrics ("potito embarrado").

146 **yips and wails of Violeta Parra:** See the introduction. A singer, composer, musician, folklorist, and visual artist, Parra was a

giant figure in the Nueva Canción movement both in Chile and throughout Latin America. She died by suicide in 1967.

146 **the star of NO:** See the introduction and chronology. A dramatized version of these events are featured in Pablo Larraín's 2012 film *No*.

147 ***todos los pobres del mundo*:** Likely referring to Quilapayún's rendition in Spanish of the communist anthem, "The Internationale."

148 ***La vida no era eterna*:** A slight misquote of "Te Recuerdo Amanda." See note on page 211–12.

148 ***En esa carta me dicen que cayó preso mi hermano*:** From the first verse of Violeta Parra's song "La carta," which begins, "They sent me a letter / By the early post / And in that letter they say / That my brother's gone to jail."

GONZALO

152 **the Concertación's victory celebrations:** La Concertación de Partidos por la Democracia (Coalition of Parties for Democracy) was founded in 1988 as a Center-Left coalition that opposed the dictatorship. Following the success of the NO campaign, the Concertación would become the dominant political force in Chile for the next two decades.

SO LONG, CHE!

156 **the brotherly rocking of *el pueblo unido jamás será vencido*:** See note above.

156 **the funeral in Havana, where even your enemies will purchase box seats:** On October 17, 1997, Cuba formally received Che's remains and interred them in a mausoleum in Santa Clara, with tens of thousands of onlookers in attendance.

DIALOGUE

159 **the same dignity that Sola Sierra had maintained for so many years:** Sola Sierra Henríquez directed the Agrupación de Familiares de Detenidos Desaparecidos (Association of Families of the Detained-Disappeared) from 1977 until her death in 1999.

160 **Volodia's son, Claudio Teitelbom:** Volodia Teitelbom was a Chilean Communist politician, lawyer, and author, who lived in exile in Moscow during the dictatorship.

161 **Viviana Díaz and Mireya García:** Díaz became president of the agrupación after Sola Sierra's death. Mireya García served as vice president.

ACT LIKE NOTHING HAPPENED, DREAM IT NEVER COULD

163 **GLORIA CAMIRUAGA'S FILM *LA VENDA*:** This crónica, first published in *Punto Final*, was written in direct response to *La venda (The blindfold)*, Camiruaga's 2000 documentary that featured interviews with women who had been tortured during the military dictatorship.

WELCOME BACK, KING TUT

167 **Augusto Nero felt the aircraft take off:** Lemebel is equating Augusto Pinochet to Nero, the Roman emperor.

167 **Merino, Leigh, and Mendoza:** Three of the five members of the original military junta. Admiral José Toribio Merino, head of the navy; General Gustavo Leigh, head of the air force; and César Mendoza Durán, general director of the police.

167 **a socialist had taken the democratic route:** The socialist in this case refers to Ricardo Lagos (b. 1938), a Chilean lawyer, economist, and politician who spoke out against the dictatorship in the 1980s and helped lead the Left's efforts during the 1988 NO campaign. He served as president from 2000 to 2006.

169 **Hospital Militar:** A high-end hospital for military personnel located in La Reina, a wealthy neighborhood at the edge of Santiago.

FINALE

ZANJÓN UPON THE WATER

175 **the bumblebee prince:** A reference to the Russian fairy tale "The Tale of Tsar Saltan."

Sources

Original publication details for all crónicas in this volume, in the order in which they appear in the book, are as follows:

"In Lieu of a Synopsis": "A modo de synopsis." *Serenata cafiola.* Santiago: Seix Barral, 2008.

MARICÓN

"Her Throaty Laugh": "Su ronca risa loca (el dulce engaño del travestismo prostibular)." *Loco afán. Crónicas de sidario.* Santiago: LOM, 1996.

"Manifesto": "Manifiesto (hablo por mi diferencia)." *Loco afán. Crónicas de sidario.* Santiago: LOM, 1996.

"Anacondas in the Park": "Anacondas en el parque." *La esquina es mi corazón. Crónica urbana.* Santiago: Cuarto Propio, 1995.

"New York Chronicles": "Crónicas de Nueva York." *Loco afán. Crónicas de sidario.* Santiago: LOM, 1996.

"Chile: Sea Men and Cueca": "Chile mar y cueca (o 'arréglate, Juana Rosa')." *La esquina es mi corazón. Crónica urbana.* Santiago: Cuarto Propio, 1995.

"Where the Music and the Lights Never Went Out": "La música y las luces nunca se apagaron." *La esquina es mi corazón. Crónica urbana.* Santiago: Cuarto Propio, 1995.

"Even Poppies Have Thorns": "Las amapolas también tienen espinas." *La esquina es mi corazón. Crónica urbana.* Santiago: Cuarto Propio, 1995.

"Wild Desire": "Loco afán." *Loco afán. Crónicas de sidario.* Santiago: LOM, 1996.

COUP

"For Five Minutes You Blossom": "Los cinco minutos te hacen florecer (Víctor Jara)." *De perlas y cicatrices. Crónicas radiales.* Santiago: LOM, 1998.

"Pisagua on Pointe": "Pisagua en puntas de pie." *Serenata cafiola.* Santiago: Seix Barral, 2008.

"If You Don't Return": "'La ciudad sin ti.'" *Serenata cafiola.* Santiago: Seix Barral, 2008.

"Merci, Beau Coup": "Las joyas del golpe." *De perlas y cicatrices. Crónicas radiales.* Santiago: LOM, 1998.

"Black Orchids": "Las orquídeas negras de Mariana Callejas (o el Centro Cultural de la DINA)." *De perlas y cicatrices. Crónicas radiales.* Santiago: LOM, 1998.

"Where Were You?": "¿Dónde estabas tú?" *Háblame de amores.* Santiago: Seix Barral, 2012.

"Ronald Wood": "Ronald Wood (a ese bello lirio despeinado)." *De perlas y cicatrices. Crónicas radiales.* Santiago: LOM, 1998.

"Night at the Circus": "Noche payasa." *Adiós mariquita linda.* Santiago: Sudamericana, 2004.

"Flash Art Politics": "La política del arte relámpago." *Háblame de amores.* Santiago: Seix Barral, 2012.

AIDS

"Diamonds Are Forever": "'Los diamantes son eternos' (frívolas, cadavéricas y ambulantes)." *Loco afán. Crónicas de sidario.* Santiago: LOM, 1996.

"Night of Furs": "La noche de los visones (o la última fiesta de la Unidad Popular)." *Loco afán. Crónicas de sidario.* Santiago: LOM, 1996.

"The Death of Madonna": "La muerte de Madonna." *Loco afán. Crónicas de sidario.* Santiago: LOM, 1996.

"Letter to Liz Taylor": "Carta a Liz Taylor (o esmeraldas egipcias para AZT)." *Loco afán. Crónicas de sidario*. Santiago: LOM, 1996.

"The Million Names of María Chameleon": "Los mil nombres de María Camaleón." *Loco afán. Crónicas de sidario*. Santiago: LOM, 1996.

"Regine, Queen of Monkey Aluminums": "La Regine de Aluminios el Mono." *Loco afán. Crónicas de sidario*. Santiago: LOM, 1996.

"Hot Pants at the Sodomy Disco": "Nalgas lycra, Sodoma Disco." *Loco afán. Crónicas de sidario*. Santiago: LOM, 1996.

"False Lashes": "Esas largas pestañas del sida local." *Loco afán. Crónicas de sidario*. Santiago: LOM, 1996.

"Loba Lamar's Last Kiss": "El último beso de Loba Lamar (crespones de seda en mi despedida . . . por favor)." *Loco afán. Crónicas de sidario*. Santiago: LOM, 1996.

POST-90

"Frou-Frou Exiles": "El exilio fru-fru (había una fonda en Montparnasse)." *De perlas y cicatrices. Crónicas radiales*. Santiago: LOM, 1998.

"The Ballad of Willy Oddó": "El rojo amanecer de Willy Oddó (o el rasguño letal de la doncella travesti)." *Loco afán. Crónicas de sidario*. Santiago: LOM, 1996.

"Aftertaste": "Chocolate amargo." *Zanjón de la Aguada*. Santiago: Seix Barral, 2003.

"Gonzalo": "Gonzalo (el rubor maquillado de la memoria)." *Loco afán. Crónicas de sidario*. Santiago: LOM, 1996.

"So Long, Che!": "Adiós al Che (o las mil maneras de despedir un mito)." *Zanjón de la Aguada*. Santiago: Seix Barral, 2003.

"Dialogue": "La Mesa de Diálogo (o el mantel blanco de una oscura negociación)." *Zanjón de la Aguada*. Santiago: Seix Barral, 2003.

"Act Like Nothing Happened, Dream It Never Could": "Hacer como que nada, soñar como que nunca (acerca del video 'La venda,' de Gloria Camiruaga)." *Zanjón de la Aguada*. Santiago: Seix Barral, 2003.

"Welcome Back, King Tut": "Bienvenido, Tutankamón (o el regreso de la pesadilla)." *Zanjón de la Aguada*. Santiago: Seix Barral, 2003.

FINALE

"Zanjón upon the Water": "Zanjón de la Aguada (crónica en tres actos)." *Zanjón de la Aguada*. Santiago: Seix Barral, 2003.

"Street Corners of My Heart": "La esquina es mi corazón (o los New Kids del Bloque)." *La esquina es mi corazón. Crónica urbana*. Santiago: Cuarto Propio, 1995.

"The Abyss of Sound": "El abismo iletrado de unos sonidos." *Adiós mariquita linda*. Santiago: Sudamericana, 2004.

"Census and the Conquest": "Censo y Conquista (¿y esa peluca rosada bajo la cama?)." *La esquina es mi corazón. Crónica urbana*. Santiago: Cuarto Propio, 1995.

"You're Mine, Girl": "Eres mío, niña." *Adiós mariquita linda*. Santiago: Sudamericana, 2004.

"The Transfiguration of Miguel Ángel": "La transfiguración de Miguel Ángel (o 'la fe mueve montañas')." *Loco afán. Crónicas de sidario*. Santiago: LOM, 1996.